To Claire with
my compliments
and love from
Aunt Clara.

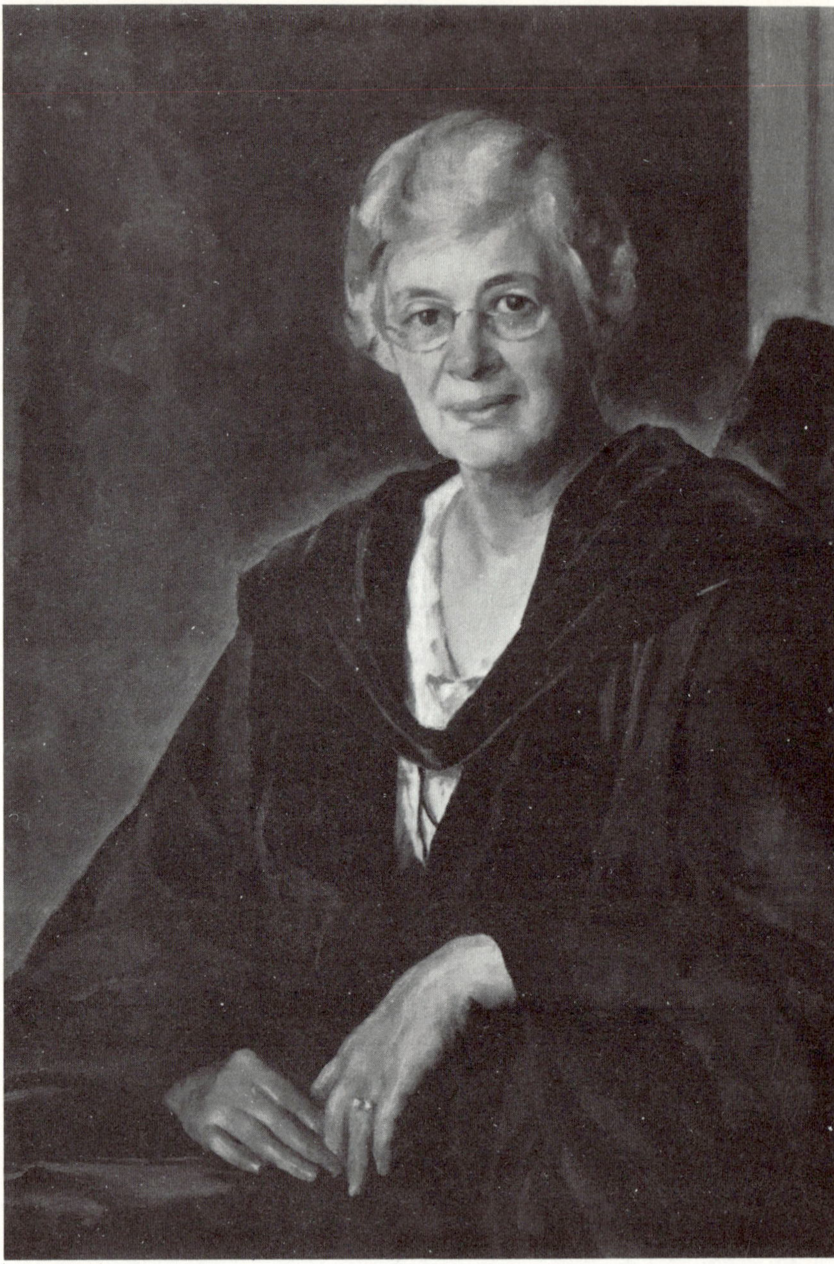

Mary Swartz Rose   1874–1941

MARY SWARTZ ROSE—1874–1941
PIONEER IN NUTRITION

MARY SWARTZ ROSE
1874-1941
PIONEER IN NUTRITION

Juanita Archibald Eagles, Ed.D.
Formerly Adjunct Professor of Nutrition
Teachers College, Columbia University

Orrea Florence Pye, Ph.D.
Professor Emeritus of Nutrition
Teachers College, Columbia University

Clara Mae Taylor, Ph.D.
Professor Emeritus of Nutrition
Teachers College, Columbia University

Clara Mae Taylor

TEACHERS COLLEGE PRESS

TEACHERS COLLEGE, COLUMBIA UNIVERSITY
NEW YORK AND LONDON

 Published by Teachers College Press,
1234 Amsterdam Avenue, New York, NY 10027.

For reprint permission, grateful acknowledgement is made to:

The American Dietetic Association for the photograph taken during the first Mary Swartz Rose Fellowship that appeared on page 1029 in Journal of the American Dietetic Association, *vol. 25, December 1949.*

Macmillan Company for Mary Swartz Rose, Feeding the Family, *1916, and third edition, 1929; and Mary Swartz Rose,* A Laboratory Handbook of Dietetics, *fourth edition, 1937.*

Library of Congress Cataloging in Publication Data

Eagles, Juanita Archibald, 1915-
Mary Swartz Rose, 1874-1941, pioneer in nutrition.

Includes bibliographies and index.
1. Rose, Mary Davies Swartz, 1874-1941.
2. Nutritionists—Biography. I. Pye, Orrea Florence, 1907- joint author. II. Taylor, Clara Mae, 1898- joint author. III. Title.
TX350.8.R67E18 613.2'092'4 [B] 79-4342
ISBN 0-8077-2556-0

Cover and Text Design: by Romeo Enriquez
Manufactured in the U.S.A.
1 2 3 4 5 6 7 8 86 85 84 83 82 81 80 79

CONTENTS

LIST OF ILLUSTRATIONS

LIST OF TABLES

FOREWORD

Biography is one of the earliest forms of literature. It is the written record of the life and personality of an individual. Biographical writing, at least for Western civilization, began with Plutarch who won enduring fame for his *Parallel Lives* in which he portrayed the character of illustrious Greeks and Romans. Through the centuries outstanding individuals in art, literature, political history, science, exploration, and other endeavors have been the subjects of biography. Carlyle has said: "Biography is by nature the most universally profitable, universally pleasant of all things: especially biography of distinguished individuals."

Curiosity is a human characteristic—curiosity about the world in which we live and about other people, especially those individuals of an earlier generation who have achieved distinction in some field of interest. This is a major reason why biographies have been written in the past and continue to be written today.

Biographies of scientists may not have as wide a popular appeal as those of public figures, but they do make a valuable contribution to the history of a particular science. This is especially true for nutrition. By diligent search in the literature, scholars and students who want to understand nutrition and its development through the years may find the research papers and related writing of the investigators in this field, thus making it possible to record the events, discoveries, and when and where the work was done. With the realization that it is in the minds of men and women that the ideas and questions for research originate, the historically minded student seeks answers to such questions as: What kind of a person was the investigator? What was the motivation to enter the field of nutrition? and What were the methods of work, problems, successes, failures, and personal interests of the research worker? This is the kind of information that biography provides, and is one reason why such writings make a significant contribution to the history of nutrition.

There have been comparatively few biographies of women in science, and this biography of Mary Swartz Rose is probably the first such book devoted to the life and work of a woman in nutrition. There are several reasons for this. Traditionally, it was firmly believed that a woman's place was in the home. Also, it was assumed that women lacked the intellectual capacity for higher education and that such pursuits would damage their health. Until the late 1800s few universities would admit women, but the establishment of the land-grant colleges opened the way for women to press their demands for education. Ellen Swallow Richards (1842–1911), who was reluctantly admitted as a special student in chemistry at Massachusetts Institute of Technology, graduated and became a successful practicing chemist, and was the founder of the American Home Economics Association (1909). She clearly demonstrated that women could succeed in science, and that their health was unimpaired by intensive study or by combining a very active professional life with that of a homemaker.

By the beginning of this century women interested in science found that nutrition was a challenging new field, and Mary Swartz Rose had the vision and capabilities to respond to that challenge. She has left her mark in the history of nutrition because she combined the intellectual abilities and human concerns to become a —

1. research worker;
2. teacher who challenged and stimulated the abilities of her students to travel with her in new pathways of thinking, observation, and practice in nutrition;
3. translator of nutrition science into practical terms for the use of homemakers and their families;
4. nutrition educator who pioneered in developing ways of teaching nutrition to boys and girls;
5. woman who had the vision to see the international implications of nutrition and to serve on the Technical Commission on Nutrition of the Health Organization of the League of Nations.

Readers of this biography will be grateful to the authors that they have undertaken the preparation of this record of the life of Mrs. Rose while those who knew her could still be consulted for their recollections.

The authors have brought to their task an intimate knowledge of the field of nutrition, and extensive research into the records, writings, letters and family history, and other resources of a biographer. They have treated all these materials with objectivity, balance, and understanding of the character and personality of their subject. Thus they have produced a volume worthy to take its place among the biographies of nutrition scientists, a source of data of historical value to scholars, and a book to provide valued information and enjoyment for all readers.

E. Neige Todhunter, Ph.D.
Visiting Professor of Nutrition
School of Medicine
Vanderbilt University

PREFACE

Mary Swartz Rose was a pioneer in nutrition and one of the pioneering professors at Teachers College, Columbia University, during the early part of the twentieth century. Colleagues have said of her that no other person contributed more to advancement in every aspect of nutrition in this century. And yet, there does not exist a complete biography of her life and work. The authors have written this volume to fill this need and to provide the story of a successful woman, researcher, teacher, and interpreter of the science of nutrition at its formative phase of development in the United States.

We believe that the biography will have value at this time when both public and private agencies are trying to develop satisfactory recommendations regarding foods and nutrition to meet today's problems. A retrospective analysis of Rose's discoveries and judgments can be helpful in the current quest for validity and practicality. The example of how one woman was able to successfully combine her private and work lives should serve as a stimulus to women seeking opportunities to expand their roles. In learning about Mary Swartz Rose we note that just recognition for women's efforts and achievements can follow from the organized and energetic career of a creative woman. The Epilogue points up the ongoing influence of such a woman. There is an increasing interest today in historical and biographical material in all fields of science, including nutrition.

The primary author, Juanita Archibald Eagles, did not know Mary Swartz Rose, but as a Teachers College person had a good background knowledge of her. In addition, she had studied undergraduate nutrition under a former student of Rose who always kept Rose's picture on her office wall and made many references to Rose's work. The coauthors, Orrea Florence Pye and Clara Mae Taylor (Mrs. Carl Olson), knew Mary Swartz Rose very well. Clara Mae Taylor had served on her staff for fourteen years. Both had been her students, had worked with her, and had access to a great deal of material written by and about Rose. Additional help in the preparation of the manuscript was obtained by the authors through interviews and correspondence with others who had known Rose.

The biography contains more than the title implies. The authors deal not only with Mary Swartz Rose but also with the institution, Teachers College, where Rose had the base and springboard for her achievements. Included is a brief history of nutrition as it influenced the career of Rose and world conditions as they related to her life and activities. Separate chapters are devoted to the evolution of her career, personal characteristics, years at Yale under Lafayette B. Mendel, teaching, research, participation in various organizations, students, and home life. A complete list of her publications is given. Also included are two Appendices. Appendix A gives an annotated list of nutrition books that were available in 1910. Appendix B lists the friends and students who participated in the Mary Swartz Anniversary Dinner in 1936.

The authors wish to acknowledge with thanks the help and encouragement given by many individuals. They especially want to express appreciation to Dr. E. Neige Todhunter who first suggested this volume and has contributed the Foreword; to all who contributed to the Epilogue; and to Mr. and Mrs. Richard C. Rose who provided access to personal correspondence and memorabilia of his parents. Although any project of this type cannot be accomplished without the help of others, the primary author assumes responsibility for any errors or omissions and thanks her collaborators for their participation.

J.A.E.
O.F.P.
C.M.T.

MARY SWARTZ ROSE—1874–1941
PIONEER IN NUTRITION

There is no instinct for a good diet. The development of habits which make for optimum nutrition is wholly a matter of education.—MSR

chapter one

MARY SWARTZ ROSE—EVOLUTION OF HER CAREER

She was able to do it because she was organized. Yes, and she had everyone else in the household organized! On her dresser there were always lists, lists for her, lists for me, lists for father and lists for the housekeeper. She really knew how to make good use of time! She and father had agreed when they were married on the duties that each would perform. Therefore mother knew exactly what her responsibilities at home were and father always said "Mary's career comes first." Mother started at her desk when father went to bed—he went to bed at ten o'clock each night because of his health and in order to be up to leave the house at six o'clock each morning—mother did not need to leave home until much later in the morning.[1]

Who was this person? Was she the modern woman of the 1970s? No, her life began a century earlier. She was Mary Swartz Rose, a key person in the development of the present knowledge of nutrition and its application, a woman who successfully combined the role of wife and mother with that of a pioneering scientist and educator.

She was born Mary Davies Swartz on October 31, 1874, in Newark, Ohio, the first of five children of Hiram B. Swartz and Martha Jane Davies Swartz (fig. 1.1). Both parents were natives of Ohio. Her father, of Dutch, German, and Scottish ancestry, was the fourth in a family of twelve children born to Samuel and Mary Swartz, pioneer farmers of Ohio. Farming for the Swartz family ended, however, because the six sons all entered the professions and the six daughters all married professional men. Her mother's family originated in Wales and came to Ohio where her mother was born, the daughter of Deacon C. Davies and Jane Davies.

Her mother had graduated from the Young Ladies Institute, which later became Shepardson College, receiving a regular Ohio State teaching license. She then taught school prior to her marriage as did her sister who had been the first woman to get teaching papers from the state of Ohio. Mrs. Swartz passed away at her daughter Mary's home during her 90th year. Martha Jane Davies Swartz was a clever, kind, efficient woman, a homemaker who was interested in public improvements and cultural affairs as well as in her home.

Hiram B. Swartz attended rural schools in Ohio and the Academy at Seville, Ohio. For a year he was a teacher in his old home school. He took a preparatory course at Denison University and then entered the law department of the University of Michigan. The following year, he entered the literary department of the University of Michigan. He graduated from both departments within the four-year period, a precedent in the history of the university. He was a member of the legal profession in Ohio until his death in his 92nd year. During that time he was president of the Wayne County Bar Association and served as probate judge of Wayne County.[2] For the last thirty years of his life Judge Swartz devoted most of his attention to patent laws. Because of his own inventive turn of mind he developed an outstanding voting machine, a washing machine, and a sash window lock.

Judge Swartz was a scholar of Latin and Greek, languages that he taught his daughter Mary who had her own Greek bible, which she read. In fact, when Mary was young she said that if she ever taught she would like to teach Greek. Judge Swartz was well read in biblical subjects. He taught Sunday school for many years and gave talks on

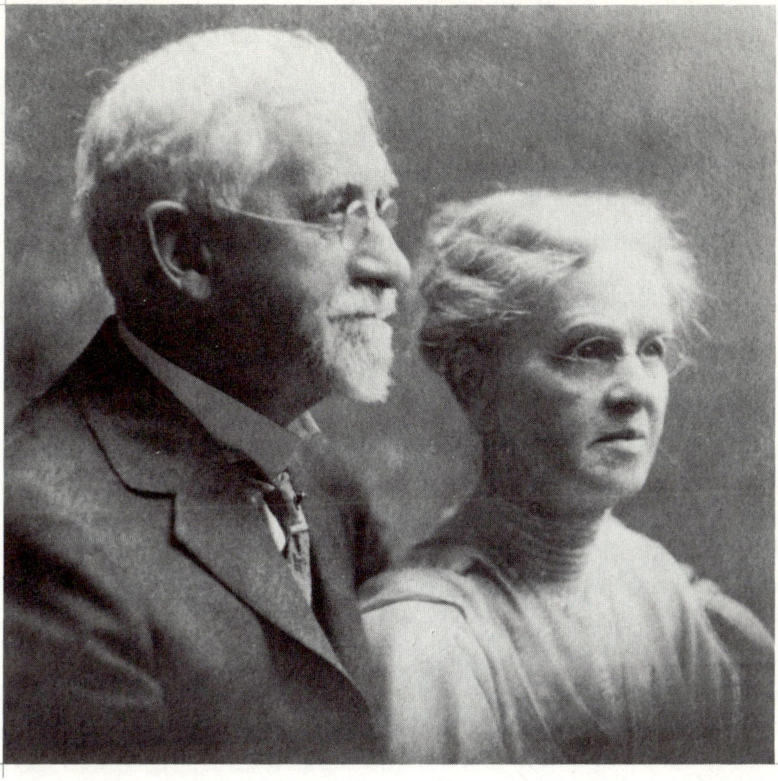

Fig. 1.1 Judge and Mrs. Hiram B. Swartz

religious subjects before many organizations. His father's family were Dunkers, that is, German Protestant refugees. When his children developed an interest in music, Judge Swartz became a Baptist and served as a deacon of his church. Later when his children became interested in dancing, he turned to the Presbyterian church, which was more liberal at that time. During his 90s, however, he was reinstated in the Baptist church from which his funeral service was held.[3]

Judge Swartz was elected mayor of Wooster, Ohio, where he had moved when Mary was three years old and where he lived until he died. During his term of office as mayor, he codified the ordinances of the city, helped in planning the installation of the first waterworks plant, and was instrumental in effecting many public improvements.

In fact, Judge Swartz was one of the city's most esteemed citizens, and was known for his boundless energy, courage, resolution, progressive ideas, and moral convictions.

Mary had two sisters and two brothers. One sister, Josephine, died in infancy and one brother, Wayne, died at a comparatively early age. The younger brother, Paul, studied engineering, married, had one daughter, Elizabeth, and made his home in Mamaroneck, New York. The younger sister, Esther, dropped the name Swartz during World War I and took the surname Davies after her mother's family. Esther Davies was in charge of Home Economics Research at the Massachusetts Agricultural Experiment Station in Amherst. She was interested in demonstrating what relationship, if any, could be found between the food habits of children of elementary school age and their state of health. In the *Agricultural Experiment Station Bulletin,* no. 241, March 1928, she wrote "The Food Consumption of Rural School Children in Relation to Their Health," and in no. 263, April 1930, "Food Service in Massachusetts Rural Elementary Schools." In the first bulletin the author acknowledged the help of her older sister Mary in the determination of scores for evaluating diets and for her kindness in reading and criticizing the manuscript.

Now that we have some understanding of her family background, let us look at Mary herself. Let us examine, from a broad viewpoint, her life and work and thereby set the stage for the subsequent story of her roles and contributions as a woman, wife, mother, scientist, educator, speaker, and writer.

From childhood Mary Davies Swartz had an attractive appearance, pleasing personality, cheerful disposition, and amiable ways. She was energetic and enthusiastic. She had the great advantage of being reared in a home that was devoted to domestic problems and improvements so that she developed scholarly and refined tastes (fig. 1.2).[4]

In her early years, she received a classical education in liberal arts. She attended the Wooster schools, graduating from high school as valedictorian of her class in 1892. She learned languages from her father, who was knowledgeable in linguistics. She studied shorthand and typing. The next nine years of her life were spent partly in Shepardson College, which was part of Denison University, Ohio, and partly in teaching history and botany in the Wooster high school. She received an Ohio State teacher's certificate in 1899 and then the

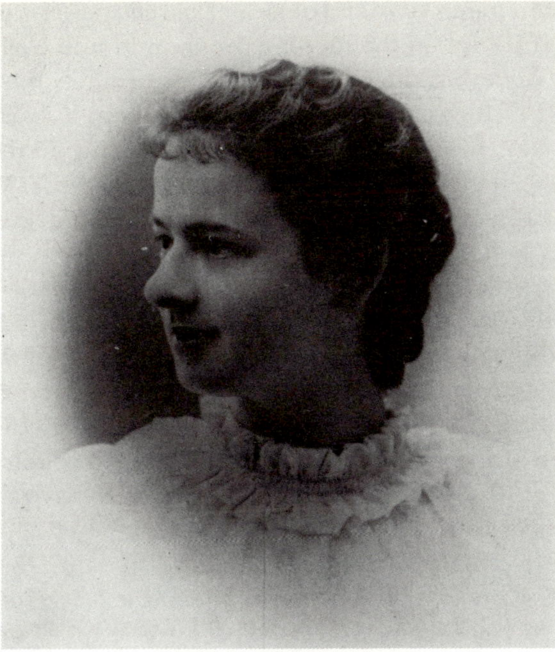

Fig. 1.2 Mary Davies Swartz as a young woman

degree of bachelor of letters from Denison University in 1901. She proved to be a young woman of unusual ability as is attested to by a review of her grades at high school and Shepardson College—an average grade of 96.5, with 19 percent of her marks 100, 29 percent 99 or 98, and less than 5 percent under 90. She then began taking courses in domestic science at Mechanics Institute, Rochester, New York, receiving a diploma in 1902. From 1902 to 1905 she taught home economics in the high school at Fond du Lac, Wisconsin.

In the autumn of 1905 she entered Teachers College, Columbia University, New York, to work toward a bachelor of science degree in chemistry at Columbia University under Professor Henry C. Sherman and a diploma in dietetics from Teachers College. She received the combined degree in 1906 while she was an assistant in dietetics at Teachers College. Her dean at Teachers College, James Earl Russell, was an educational administrator who encouraged female leaders. He granted Mary Swartz a traveling fellowship in 1907 to study physiological chemistry at Yale University under Professor Lafayette B. Mendel, who was a personal friend of Dean Russell and who gave encouragement and advice on the training program in nutrition developing at Teachers College. Professor Mendel was a source of inspiration to Mary Swartz throughout her entire life—she kept his photograph on her desk. Mary Swartz was elected to membership in the Society of Sigma Xi, the first woman ever so honored by the Yale University chapter. She was awarded the doctor of philosophy degree by Yale in 1909.

In the autumn of 1909 Dr. Mary Swartz came back to Teachers College, as the first full-time person in the United States to develop a program in nutrition. She planned and equipped the first laboratory to be devoted solely to the training of students in nutrition and developed a training program in nutrition and dietetics. Her extraordinary scholarship and success in teaching were recognized by rapid promotion. In 1910 she became the first woman to have a professorial appointment in nutrition in the United States.

While at Yale Mary Swartz met a fellow student, Anton Richard Rose, who had an adjoining bench in one of the laboratories but who spoke little to her beyond "Please pass the test tube" or some such remark. At Christmas time, however, he placed a small Christmas tree on her bench, a tree decorated with a diamond ring from the five and ten cent store. Such was his proposal of marriage!

Anton R. Rose was born in Marine, Minnesota, February 22, 1877. His paternal and maternal great-grandparents and grandparents had been among the earliest settlers in Minnesota, coming from Smoland, Sweden. His father had adopted the surname "Rose" in place of his Swedish surname "Gabrielson."

Anton Rose attended Gustavus Adolphus College, Minnesota, and later the school of chemistry at Minnesota University from which he received the bachelor of science degree in 1904. He then worked in the department of chemistry at the New Hampshire College of Agriculture and Mechanic Arts. In 1906 he worked in the department of chemistry of the New York Agricultural Experiment Station from which he received a nine-month leave of absence to study at Yale University. He received the master of science degree in physiological chemistry from Yale in 1911.

Anton Rose came to Columbia University in 1910 as an assistant in the department of biological chemistry at the College of Physicians and Surgeons and continued his graduate studies, receiving the doctor of philosophy in biological chemistry in 1912. He continued doing research at Columbia while he was teaching at Fordham University, where he was professor of chemistry from 1920 to 1924. He became chief chemist of the Prudential Insurance Company and, shortly before his retirement from the company, head of the medical department. He died on September 23, 1948.

Mary Davies Swartz and Anton Richard Rose were married on September 15, 1910. Grace MacLeod, a friend and associate, said that "Theirs was a beautiful companionship marked by mutual devotion which deepened and strengthened with the years."[5]

Richard Collin Rose, their only child, was born in 1915. He graduated from Middlebury College, Vermont, and did his graduate work at Yale University, receiving the master of forestry degree in 1940. During his boyhood he spent many summers with his Swartz grandparents. Shortly after his mother's death, he was introduced to his future wife, Marjorie Paine Mitchell, by his cousin Elizabeth. Mr. and Mrs. Richard C. Rose now live in a beautiful mountainside home in Rutland, Vermont. They have one son Richard Mitchell Rose, one daughter Kristine Ann Bourassa (Mrs. J. Jerome Bourassa), and four grandchildren, Stephen Andrew Rose, Wendy Susan Rose, Todd James Bourassa, and Mark David Bourassa (fig. 1.3).

In 1920 Anton and Mary Swartz Rose made their home in Edgewater, New Jersey. She had a lovely garden where she grew many beautiful flowers—especially pink roses. Their home was a center of gracious hospitality shared with her students and with their many friends and associates. She lived there until her untimely death, February 2, 1941, at 66 years of age. Her funeral service was held at Riverside Church with the pastor, Harry Emerson Fosdick, conducting the service. She had been a member of this church for the last years of her life and attended services each Sunday. She was buried in Granville, Ohio.

Henry C. Sherman said that Mary Swartz Rose exemplified perfectly the definition of what the modern doctorate should mean: "A broadly educated person sharpened to a point."[6] As a professor of nutrition, she was first of all a scientific worker. She contributed to the development of all the major aspects of nutrition—energy, protein, mineral elements, and vitamin values. Through her research she advanced knowledge of many types of food—cereals, bread, milk, vegetables, fruits, and nuts. She was responsible for the development

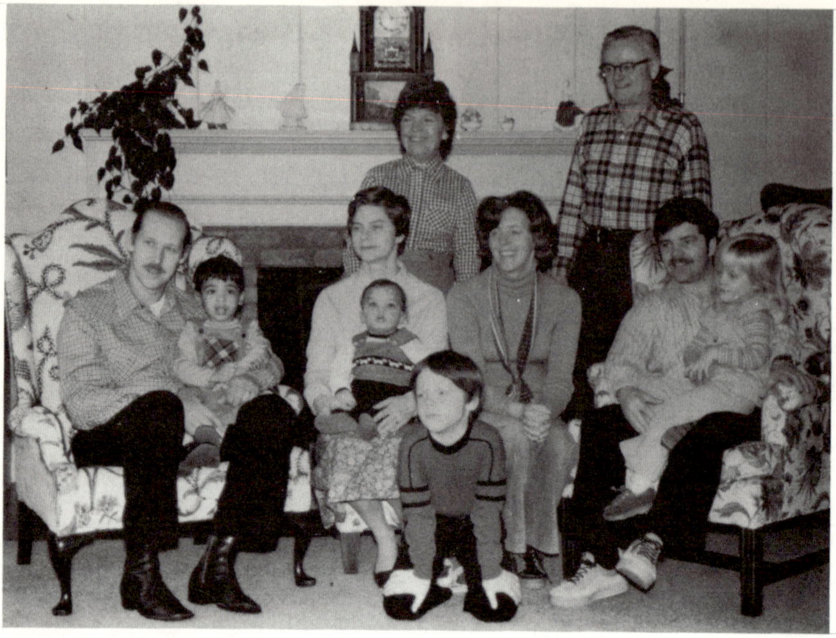

Fig. 1.3 Mr. and Mrs. Richard C. Rose with their children and grandchildren—left to right: seated, *J. Jerome Bourassa with Todd James Bourassa on his lap; Kristine Ann Bourassa with Mark David Bourassa on her lap;* kneeling, *Stephen Andrew Rose;* standing, *Mrs. Richard C. Rose;* seated, *Janet B. Rose;* standing, *Richard C. Rose;* seated, *Richard M. Rose with Wendy Susan Rose on his lap*

of the science of nutrition as an independent field separate from physiology and biological chemistry. Other scientists were also interested in building a science of nutrition out of the existing multitude of fragments of knowledge and joined together to found the prestigious society now known as the American Institute of Nutrition (AIN) in 1928. Mary Swartz Rose had the distinction of being the only woman among the eleven illustrious so-called Founding Fathers of AIN.[7] She was a member of the original board of directors of the institute, served on the editorial board of its *Journal of Nutrition,* and then became president of AIN in 1937, the first woman to hold that office.

Mary Swartz Rose was recognized as a gifted and successful teacher. She inspired the development of latent capacities in her students. Among her greatest contributions were the people she discovered, trained, and stimulated through her teaching to the highest order of professional and social service in the food and nutrition field. Her students felt personal affection and admiration for her and were continually surprised by her range of interests. A student of 1912–13 recalls that she dismissed class early one day so that the students could watch the suffrage parade down Fifth Avenue led by Inez Milholland riding a beautiful white horse. Mary Swartz Rose believed that women would have the right to vote someday and she wanted her students to be responsible citizens.[8]

Another aspect of her work in addition to research and teaching was that of carrying nutrition directly into public service. It was said of her in 1939 that she was the strongest living link between the laboratory and the consumer of food.[9] She has been called "a democratic scientist" because she devoted her life to acquiring knowledge needed to improve the health of every man, woman, and child.[10] She believed in establishing sound food policies for everybody and putting those food policies within the reach of the average person. She extended the science of nutrition to the public through her work in local, national, and international agencies and through her writings. She wrote a number of books: *A Laboratory Handbook for Dietetics* for nutrition major students, published in 1912 and revised in 1921, 1929, and 1937; *Feeding the Family* for mothers and homemakers, published in 1916 and revised in 1924, 1929, and 1940, which has been identified as a classic in nutrition and dietetics;[11]*Foundations of Nutrition* for non-nutrition major students, published in 1927 and revised in 1933 and 1938; and in 1932 *Teaching Nutrition to Boys and Girls* for elementary school teachers. She also wrote many monographs, research papers, and addresses. (For a complete list of publications, see page 152).

She found time to take an active part in many important scientific and professional organizations, as in AIN already mentioned. She was invited to serve as a member of the Committee (now Council) on Foods and Nutrition of the American Medical Association and as a member, the only woman from the United States, on the international Technical Commission on Nutrition of the Health Organization of the League of Nations. The American Dietetic Association conferred on her their honorary membership[12] and, after her death, established a fellowship in her name (fig. 1.4).[13] (For a complete list of honors and memberships, see chapter 8).

In 1935 the international quarterly, *Nutrition Abstracts and Reviews,*

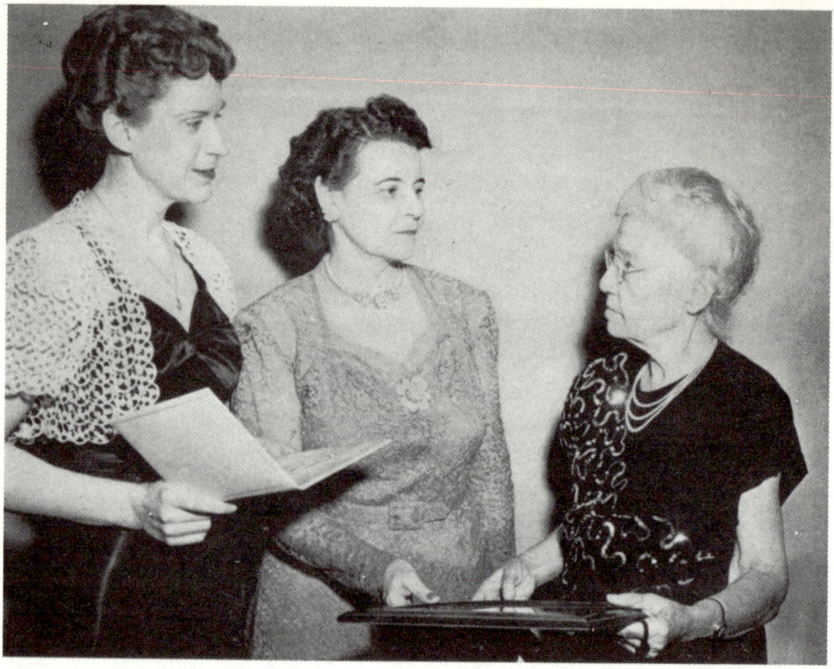

Fig. 1.4 At the banquet of the American Dietetic Association (1949), Pearl Jackson holds the portfolio that Dr. Clara Mae Taylor presented to her as the first Mary Swartz Rose Fellow. On the right, *Fairfax Proudfit, recipient of the fifth Marjorie Hulsizer Copher Award, is seen with the framed scroll that explains her signal recognition. (Courtesy of the American Dietetic Association)*

chose her to review and interpret the development of college and university teaching of nutrition and dietetics in the United States. In the same year she was named as one of the twenty-five American women to achieve international recognition in their professions. She was the first woman to receive the annual award of distinction of the Associated Grocery Manufacturers of America. During World War I she served as deputy director of conservation in the Food Administration, and in 1940 she was appointed as one of a group of advisers on nutrition to the Council of National Defense. Hers was a world-wide influence resulting from a combination of effectiveness and versatility due partly to her innate gifts, partly to the inspiration she received from Professor Mendel, and partly to the self-discipline that made her the personification of sincerity and an exemplar of the spirit of science.[14]

She had an infinite capacity for hard work. Her husband, in speaking of her energy during a discussion of the question of careers for married women, said "Well, I'm glad my wife has a career. I shouldn't like to have her expend all the energy she has just on me."[15]

> Only by working with maximum efficiency and economy of time and energy could one accomplish all she did in the short span of 66 years. She made every minute count, whether at work or play, and reaped the results of a rich, full life. . . . She could turn from exacting scientific research to preparations for a party in her home, the games and refreshments for which were the products of her ingenuity and her deftness in cookery, or to plans for improvements in her house and garden, or to teaching her dog some new tricks, or to making a dress or hat, or to going to the theatre or a movie for recreation with husband and son—all with a zest and vigor and such manifold results that it is small wonder that Dr. Mendel once said of her, "You know Arnold Benedict has written a book on *How to Live on Twenty-Four Hours a Day*. Well, Mrs. Rose has beaten him—she has found the twenty-fifth hour."[16]

Faith without works is as ineffectual in nutrition as in religion.—MSR

chapter two CHARACTERISTICS OF ROSE

What was she really like? Many people of genius are complicated human beings whose complexities puzzle the biographer. With Mary Swartz Rose there is not the problem of the many-faceted personality of opposing qualities that vary with time and place. All who knew her are in general agreement as to her personal characteristics—those referred to most frequently are her integrity, her sincerity, her vivacity, her charm.

There are many photographs and her portrait to show her physical characteristics—as a child (fig. 2.1), and later throughout life since photography was a hobby of her husband. She was a person of small stature, only about five feet in height and scarcely tipping the scales at one hundred pounds, but of arresting appearance due to her dignity, handsome features, and dark sparkling eyes that could be sharp and penetrating or twinkling with mirth.[1] She was very feminine in appearance. She always wore dresses, usually of colored floral design, never suits, which she considered too masculine. She made many of her own clothes and took pleasure in trimming her own hats. She always liked to be "dressed in style" or a little ahead if possible. One of the features that she liked about her portrait wearing the academic gown (frontispiece) was that it would never go out of style![2]

If there was no serious problem occupying her attention, she turned to everyday situations. She commuted each day from her

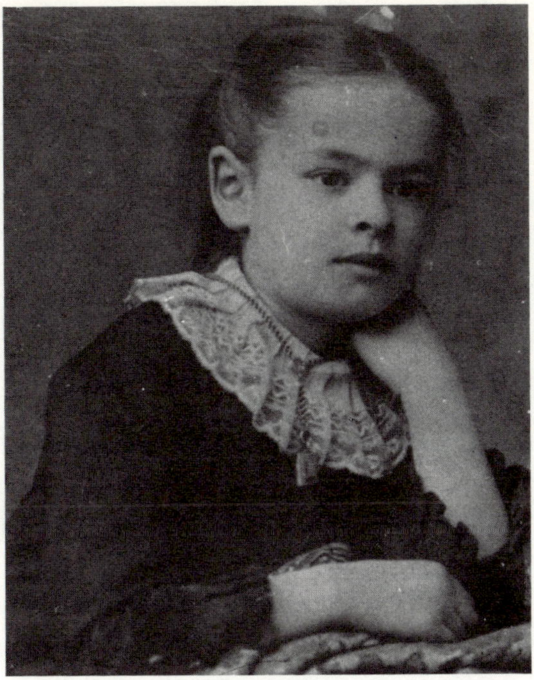

Fig. 2.1 Mary Davies Swartz as a child

home in Edgewater, New Jersey, by ferryboat to 125th Street in Manhattan, and walked or took the trolley to the college. She frequently brought in interesting tales of the people she met each day on the ferry, and delighted in making unexpected comments. One morning she came into the office with the statement that "she had figured out that she had spent more time on the Edgewater Ferry than Noah had spent on the Ark."[3]

She was alert and quick. She walked with a rapid gait. Her motions were swift and purposeful, never nervous or futile. Her whole body seemed to have controlled energy. In her youth she was quite athletic, and did a lot of riding, ice skating, dancing; in later life she walked about a mile each day, often with her dog Don Marquis, (fig. 2.2). She had an infectious smile and a joyous sort of laughter (fig. 2.3). She has been described as a sprite.

One had the impression that there was always something on her mind—the next thing to do or to plan. One had to learn to work with Mary Swartz Rose because she was a very fast thinker. She would

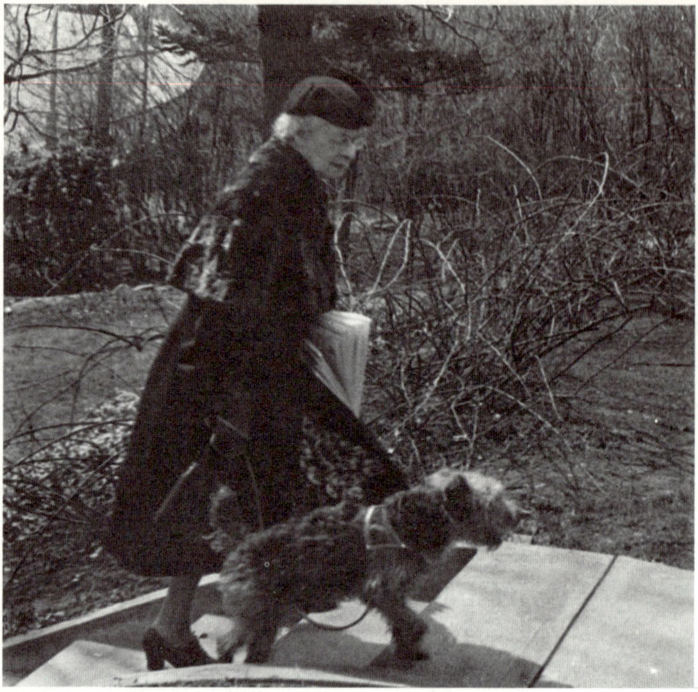

Fig. 2.2 Mary Swartz Rose with her dog Don Marquis

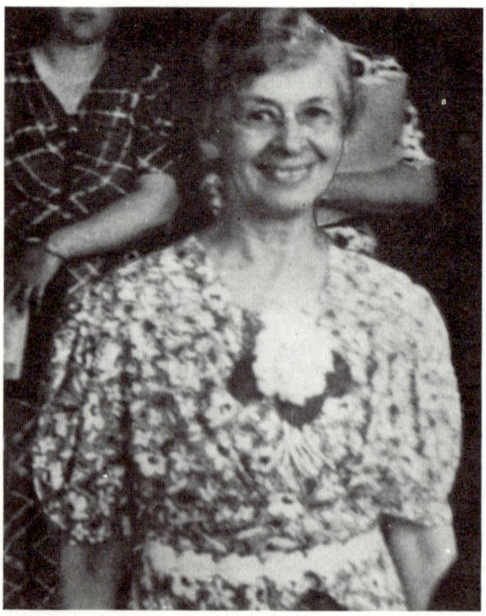

Fig. 2.3 "An infectious smile"

start a thought but not finish it, expecting the listener to fill in and understand, and she would move on to the next idea.[4]

She had great powers of concentration and a very retentive mind. She could pick up a subject, work on it, drop it, and then pick it up again without lack of continuity. Students felt the spell of her mind and sometimes were in awe of her at first but soon were stimulated to do their best.[5] She never imposed her ideas upon others. She encouraged people to develop ideas, and they often reached goals that they never expected to be able to reach. She had the ability for making everybody work.

Mary Swartz Rose had an analytical temperament, initiative, and perseverance. As Sherman once said of her with a chuckle commenting on her performance in the student seminar, "She was never satisfied with the time of day, but had to look at the inside of a watch to find out what made it tick." She was well disciplined and had a great sense of responsibility. She had high standards of performance, and, although patient with people generally, could become impatient if they failed to meet her expectations. She rarely became angry, but when she did, it was with due provocation. She flared quickly. As a former student reports:

> I taught dietetics at . . . College plus various other courses. I sometimes appealed to Mrs. Rose for help. Dietetics was in the School of Education and one time the Dean challenged my credentials to teach. I quoted my teaching at Teachers College and reported it to Mrs. Rose. She wrote a stinging letter to the Dean and sent me a carbon copy.[6]

She had great loyalty to country, family, friends, and any group to which she belonged. She did not criticize people, and one could not tell by look or comment whether she agreed with criticisms that others were making. She was interested in world affairs and in politics. In a letter (November 8, 1918) to her husband who was serving his country as a captain in the Sanitary Corps, she wrote:

> New York has had its peace celebration. I suppose that every one in the United States knows that New York City went wild a little bit previously yesterday. It is comforting to think that the day for the genuine celebration is certainly not far off. . . . I left the College at one o'clock and the whistles on the boats in the River were just beginning to blow. The New York Central train went steaming up the shore with the whis-

> tle on full blast. When I got to the Food Board, I saw the funniest sight I have seen in a long time—a group of the Food Board men standing around the door, celebrating peace with the most doleful countenances imaginable. They looked like the chief mourners at a funeral. This was because the same paper which announced the signing of the armistice had also announced the election of Smith [as governor of New York State]. Today the election is as uncertain as the signing of the armistice.[7]

Although Mary Swartz Rose accomplished so much, she never seemed worried or to be under pressure. She once said that her mother had told her to do the most important thing first and not worry about other things. She followed this precept with success. As her sister-in-law wrote:

> Another thing that stands out when I think of her is her orderliness and poise. Many times I have found her with work piled up clamoring to be done, but it never seemed to make for confusion—she always knew what must be done next and could even take time out for a friend or to do a needed kindness.[8]

She combined thrift and generosity. She enjoyed a bargain but never held on to her money when someone's need or pleasure called for it.[9] If she felt that someone was in need, she followed it up and did something about it. As is reported:

> When Mrs. . . . was old and destitute (in the 1930's), former pupils and friends started a pension fund for her. Mary Swartz Rose was a regular subscriber.[10]

She believed that one of the most important learnings for a student is how to get along with other people. She exemplified this belief. She had great insight into human nature and the capacity for putting herself in another's place. Combined with this were her unfailing kindness and friendliness and utter lack of affectation. She remembered the little things. She was interested in the student or colleague as a person. She enjoyed seeing how other people did everyday tasks. One of her great strengths was her ability to make people feel at ease and then work with them even though they had different backgrounds, abilities, and allegiances.

> She was a comfortable house guest—considerate and ready for any fun. She seemed to visit with our simple people as easily as with her Columbia colleagues; perhaps she appreciated fine quality in people wherever she found it. My aunts had never seen a college nor read books on nutrition and were hesitant about cooking for Mary, but hospitality demanded that Anton's wife must be entertained and that meant, to them, food and much food. Mary appreciated their good cooking even if there was too much of it, and they soon forgot the Ph.D. professor of nutrition and had as good a time with their new niece as if they had always known her.
>
> An incident that summer which we enjoyed might illustrate both her fun and kindliness. Her hostess at a reception for her served coffee. Since Mary did not drink coffee that was a problem, but seemingly she sipped her coffee as she moved about visiting with guests and even came back to her hostess for a second cup. She really drank very little of it and, when chance favored us, she emptied most of her coffee into my cup and went back to sipping coffee and chatting with some late coming guests. No one was the wiser. Both kindly hostess and we were happy.[11]

Mary Swartz Rose had inherent artistic qualities. She was interested in art and kept up to date on the current exhibits. She enjoyed music throughout life; as a girl she played the guitar and sang. In literature, her tastes ran from the factual and abstract masters to light reading if it were cleverly whimsical. She herself liked to write amusing verse and prose. She preferred Henry and William James, Henry Adams, Ibsen, Willa Cather, A. A. Milne, and Lewis Carroll.[12] She was a very rapid reader, frequently reading quickly first for content and then slowly, and sometimes aloud, for the flow of words and phrases. She would read a textbook as one would a novel! She was a scholar of the Bible and interested in Chinese literature.

She was a stimulating person to have about—interested in everything, a lovely sense of humor, always ready for fun.[13] She could talk entertainingly and with knowledge on almost any subject. She was a happy, pleasant person even while serious, a dynamic and at the same time gentle person.[14]

In her writings, she took the attitude that nothing was ever so good that it could not be improved. She welcomed suggestions and the opinions of others to which she gave serious consideration, but she never wanted to be told what to do. She often had her pages retyped many times, hoping that each time what she wrote would be more interesting, clearer, and the selection of words more to her satisfaction. She considered this the test of good writing, and that it was her privilege to change her mind. In this respect she was certainly a perfectionist.

She never appreciated anyone predicting her reaction to a question, and strongly protested against the idea of anyone thinking that she could be pigeonholed.

She was careful not to monopolize a conversation, and encouraged others to tell their stories. Even if she had heard the story before, she listened attentively with interest and enthusiasm. She enjoyed telling jokes on herself.

Her unusual mind was always active, and we can surmise that much of her creative thinking was done when she was engaged in chores about the house, gardening, or clearing out her files at the college. She often took on this last task when it seemed that the pressures on her time were greatest. It seemed to help clear her mind when she could weed out that which had no value and save that which had great promise for the future.

It was both a challenge and great fun working with Mary Swartz Rose. In teaching with her, it was like working on a play. She never went to class unprepared no matter how many times she had taught the same lesson—the new developments were always discussed and decisions made on how they could be interpreted to enrich the particular lesson. In working with her on her books or in trying to find answers to the many questions arriving in her daily mail, she gave undivided attention. When she reached a point at which her thoughts seemed to be approaching a standstill, she would say, "Let's stop and have a picnic." Then she and her colleagues would take the ferry to Edgewater, pick up her husband, the car, and the ever-ready picnic kit. Off they would go to a nearby picnic area. The soup kettle and the handy sterno were quickly put in service along with provisions from the refrigerator.

Speaking more than half a century ago, Rose considered good nutrition one of the most fundamental of modern problems, and this is still true today. She was truly a pioneer in a world that knew little about the principles of good nutrition. She considered better nutrition to be one of the most important of our tools to bring the greatest happiness and usefulness to the greatest number of people. She visualized a land in which men and women, boys and girls, would be happy, healthy, and wholesome. She was dedicated to a cause—that of promoting better nutrition for everyone worldwide—and she never lost sight of this goal.

Nutrition deals with the scientific laws governing the requirements of human beings for maintenance, growth, activity, reproduction, and lactation.—MSR

chapter three THE YEARS AT YALE UNIVERSITY

SOME HISTORICAL NOTES

Although nutrition is called a twentieth century science, the story of nutrition goes back through the centuries and is as old as the story of humans. Primitive people ate foods to survive—they were hunters of wild animals and gatherers of wild plants. They learned to domesticate animals, raise crops, and cook food. From early drawings on the wall of a tomb in the Great Pyramid of Cheops there are scenes representing the grinding of grains and the making of bread, the slaughtering and cooking of domesticated animals and poultry, the brewing of beer, and the playing of music while the master ate.[1]

Early concepts in nutrition were philosophical rather than scientific. Hippocrates (460–370 B.C.) was the philosopher most interested in food. He has been called the father of medicine. He attributed the development of medical knowledge to the problems of nutrition, for he wrote:

> To me it appears . . . that nobody would have sought for medicine at all, provided the same kinds of diet had suited with men in sickness as in good health.[2]

Several of Hippocrates' famous aphorisms dealt with nutrition; for example:

> Growing bodies have the most innate heat; they therefore require the most food for otherwise their bodies are wasted. In old people the heat is feeble and they require little fuel. . . .[3]

The term "innate heat" endured for many centuries. But for about two thousand years Hippocrates and his successors accounted for the disappearance of food as "insensible perspiration" and "heat" without any real understanding of what either term meant. Galen (130–200 A.D.), who after Hippocrates is considered the greatest medical person of ancient times, believed that the heart was the source of innate heat.

After the fall of the Greek and Roman empires, people were intellectually dependent on the heritage of the past civilizations. Not enough new facts were discovered to bring about new ideas until the fifteenth century when men once again became critics and independent investigators. Leonardo da Vinci (1452–1519), who has been called the father of modern sciences, believed that life like the flame of a candle is dependent on nutrition and that where there is life there is heat.[4] The Italian physiologist, Sanctorius (1561–1636), who devised a chair connected with a steelyard to weigh himself before and after meals, spent most of his life trying to determine the amount of "insensible perspiration" lost from his body. But his painstaking efforts did not solve the mystery, and there was no science of chemistry then to help him.[5]

It was not until the seventeenth century when investigations of the properties of air were carried out that the exact science of chemistry began and an understanding of what happens to food in the body developed.

In 1660 Robert Boyle (1627–91) demonstrated the dependence of animals upon the air they breathe for life. John Mayow (1643–79) was the first to recognize, in 1668, that breathing brings air into contact with the blood. In 1754 Joseph Black (1728–99) identified "fixed air," which he found extinguished a candle flame. He discovered that animals expired "fixed air" and concluded that the breathing of animals changed "common air" into "fixed air."

Both Joseph Priestley (1733–1804) and Karl Scheele (1742–86) independently discovered the same new gas at about the same time. Since there was no pressure for rapid publication in those days, Scheele's work, which was discovered first, was not published until after Priestley s. Priestley is therefore given credit for the discovery of the new gas in 1774, which he called "dephlogisticated air." This gas caused a candle to burn more brightly, and when a person inhaled it, "his breath felt peculiarly light and easy for some time afterward."[6] Scheele in 1771 had called his new gas "fire air." Priestley lost favor in England due to his support of the French revolutionists, fled to the United States, and lived in Northumberland, Pennsylvania, until his death. His home, in which his laboratory was located, has been preserved as a lasting memorial to Priestley.

Both Priestley and Scheele were in communication with a young French nobleman, Antoine Laurent Lavoisier (1743–94). Lavoisier repeated their experiments at their requests and confirmed the discovery that "fixed air" was carbon dioxide. He gave the name oxygen to Priestley's and Scheele's gas. He showed that oxygen is converted to carbon dioxide in the lungs, and that respiration is only the process of slow combustion in the body. He demonstrated that animal heat is derived from oxidation within the body. Lavoisier was highly respected as a scientist because he interpreted the knowledge of the time and added his own findings to the field of chemistry. He had political problems, however, and was beheaded by the French revolutionists at 51 years of age. Because of his grasp of the respiratory process in relation to food, Lavoisier is called the father of the science of nutrition.[7]

Thus, by the end of the eighteenth century, scientific concepts formed the basis of nutrition knowledge. And although conditions of the times were right for continued expansion of scientific knowledge, progress in the new science of nutrition was slow. Nutrition had to wait for developments in various other sciences. What Lavoisier had learned about combustion was not applied immediately to physiology. That remained the task of the nineteenth century scientists.

Justus von Liebig (1803–73), who is called the first organic chemist, was the first to understand that the substances oxidized for fuel in the body are organic compounds of three types—carbohydrates, fats, and proteins. He emphasized the fact that the same substances occur in our foods and as constituents of our bodies, and that the latter arise from the former.[8] He not only created organic chemistry but also extended it to physiology and agriculture.[9] Pupils came to Liebig from all over the world. They became leaders in the physiology of metabolism and nutrition.

Carl von Voit (1831–1908) was Liebig's most famous pupil. Voit graduated in medicine after the usual six years of study. He then began advanced study in physics, zoology, anatomy, and in chemistry under Liebig, who became his lifelong inspiration. Voit's chemistry laboratory desk was next to that of an American, George J. Brush, who later became famous as the first director of the Sheffield Scientific School, Yale University. Voit, with the cooperation of Max von Pettenkofer, constructed a respiration chamber and studied energy and protein metabolism in dogs and men. Among other findings, Voit demonstrated that nitrogen of the feces and urine could be used as a measure of protein metabolism in an animal, that carbohydrate reduces the amount of protein necessary for nitrogen equilibrium, and that muscular work is not done at the expense of protein. Voit is reported to have said to his pupils early in their courses, "You need not believe anything of what I relate to you in my lectures, you need only believe what I can demonstrate and prove to you."[10]

Now let us consider three of Voit's pupils. First, Max Rubner (1854–1932) and then two who were from the United States, namely Graham Lusk (1866–1932) and Wilbur O. Atwater (1844–1907). Rubner, one hundred years after its initial conception by Lavoisier, established by animal experimentation the fundamental law that energy is neither created nor destroyed in the body. He further extended understanding of energy metabolism in the body and the energy values of foods. He gave us the familiar calorie values of food—4, 9, and 4 calories per gram of protein, fat, and carbohydrate respectively. Lusk became a distinguished scientist, first at Yale University and later in New York. He developed a calorimeter in the Cornell Medical School and, along with E. F. DuBois, calorimeters at Bellevue Hospital in New York City and at the New York Hospital. Lusk pioneered in research in metabolic studies in humans and animals. He was a critical, objective thinker—he wrote from the viewpoint of his own research and the publications of other scientists in order to synthesize the then current knowledge. His book, *Science of Nutrition,* dedicated to Voit and published in 1906, was one of the first to show the scientific basis of nutrition. It was used through subsequent revisions as a text for several decades; undoubtedly, it was used by Mary Swartz in her graduate studies at Yale. Atwater designed with his research partners the first calorimeter to be used for human nutrition research in the United States; published the first analysis of an American food (corn) in 1869; and in 1896 he and his associates at the United States Department of Agriculture published the first edition of the agriculture bulletin containing tables showing the composition of familiar foods—bulletin 28. This bulletin was the basis of all dietary studies and dietetic work in the United States for many years. Atwater has been referred to as the father of American nutrition.[11]

There are many bypaths in the history of nutrition that might have been followed. We have briefly reviewed the path that led through the eras of philosophical and scientific concepts of metabolism to the beginning of the twentieth century, a time when energy and calories were of prime interest and importance. By then nutrition was an established science, based on chemistry and physiology. Knowledge in nutrition had expanded from the one universal and unchangeable aliment of Hippocrates to the multiple-nutrient concept—carbohydrates, fats, proteins, and certain minerals. Very little was known, however, about the role of minerals in nutrition. Iron, calcium, phosphorus, potassium, sulfur, sodium, chlorine, and magnesium were known to exist in the body in measurable amounts. Vitamins were unknown; in fact, the word had not yet been coined. There was little understanding of the relation of foods to health.[12]

THE SHEFFIELD SCIENTIFIC SCHOOL, YALE UNIVERSITY

The first definitive laboratory of physiological chemistry in America for the instruction of students was established in the Sheffield Scientific School in 1874.[13] Russell H. Chittenden (1856–1943) was placed in charge of it and taught a small group of students in 1874, when he was only eighteen years old. He became professor of physiological chemistry in 1882. His research interests in nutrition were in protein metabolism, especially in minimal protein requirements of healthy males. He had wide research interests in other areas also; for example, he was one of the first American scientists to study the chemistry of the brain.[14]

Lafayette B. Mendel (1872–1935) was Chittenden's best pupil. When Chittenden succeeded Brush as director of the Sheffield Scientific School in 1898, Mendel took over the supervision of graduate students and much of the teaching. Chittenden continued to give a course in nutrition each year, a subject in which he was deeply interested, and a course in toxicology. Thus, graduate students had intimate contact with both of these men of superior talents.

The physiological chemistry laboratory in those years was very stimulating. Mendel was at the height of his powers, intensely enthusiastic, studious, and a great teacher.[15] Mendel was probably the greatest single influence in the scientific life of his students.[16] It was said that at that time no one anywhere surpassed Mendel in thoroughness of instruction in biochemistry, a fact supported by the long list of his students who gained distinction as teachers and investigators.[17] In fact, until about 1915 a large proportion of the biochemists in this country had their training at Yale.[18] During his relatively short career Mendel published three hundred thirty papers; ninety-two students received the Ph.D. degree under his direction; two hundred thirty-seven graduate students and ninety-two research fellows and visitors acquired part of their training under his influence.[19] Mendel is known for his early studies on vitamins, and for his constant consideration of the organism as a whole. Mendel and T. B. Osborne are especially known for their work on proteins and amino acids on which they published over one hundred papers.

Elmer V. McCollum recalled that Chittenden, Mendel, and F. P. Underhill (assistant professor of physiological chemistry) made no mention of beriberi, scurvy, rickets, or pellagra in their 1906–07 classes. Mendel's instruction was based to a great extent on the researches of Voit, Pettenkofer, Rubner, Atwater, Lusk, and Pavlov, but everything known about metabolic processes was set before his students.[20]

MARY SWARTZ'S CLASSMATES AT YALE, 1908

Mary Swartz was a member of a group of eleven students in 1907–08 (fig. 3.1). There was only one other woman in the class, Edna L. Ferry. Apparently there was some discrimination practiced against women since the nine men in the class formed an informal social group called the Lobsters that went out together once a month for dinner and an evening of celebration. Women of the laboratory were known as Snails, and were banned from membership in the Lobsters. The Lobsters were Stanley R. Benedict, George E. Gage, Warren W.

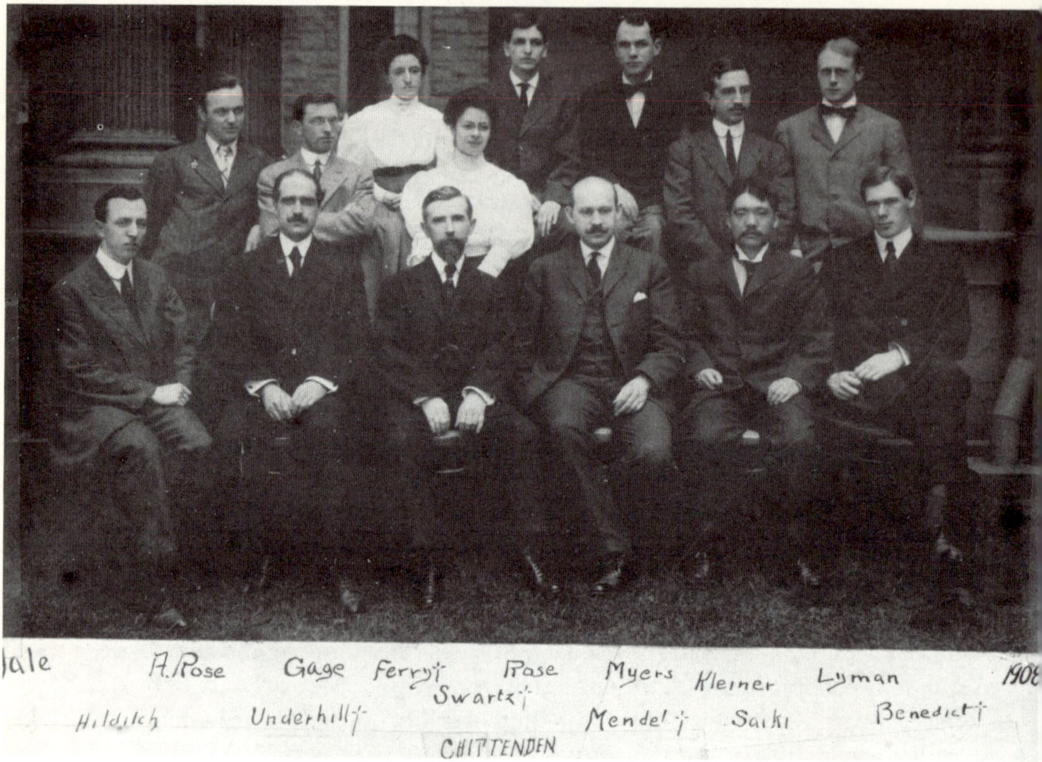

Fig. 3.1 Sheffield Scientific School, Yale University, 1908

Hilditch, Israel S. Kleiner, John F. Lyman, Victor C. Myers, Tadasu Saiki, Anton R. Rose, and William C. Rose.

While a member of this student group Mary Swartz felt that she had to compete, rather unfairly, with males who could get along with much less sleep than she![21] In later life, as mentioned in chapter 1, she too learned how to reduce her hours of sleep in order to reach her goals. Sleepy she was not—she did well at Yale. She was elected to Sigma Xi in 1909, the first woman member of the Yale chapter. Election to Sigma Xi was a much desired prize at Yale. She became a member of the American Association for the Advancement of Science in 1908 and of the Connecticut Academy of Arts and Sciences in 1909. She received the Ph.D. degree in physiological chemistry in 1909 (fig. 3.2).

Edna L. Ferry (1883–1919) was a graduate of Mt. Holyoke College. She was the first woman to receive the M.S. degree from Yale (1913) while on the staff of the Research Laboratory of Connecticut Agricultural Experiment Station, where she remained until her death. Her essay, "The Rate of Growth in the Albino Rat," was published in *Anatomical Record,* vol. 7, 1913.

Ferry wrote "The Value of Milk" as a bulletin of the Connecticut Agricultural Experiment Station, which was reprinted in various forms and translated into French. She also wrote two papers in cooperation with Osborne and Mendel: "The Effect of Retardation of Growth upon the Breeding Period and Duration of Life of Rats" (*Science,* vol. 45, 1917) and "A Method of Expressing Numerically the Growth-Promoting Value of Proteins" (*Journal of Biological Chemistry,* vol. 37, 1919); and one with Osborne and A. J. Wakeman "Prepara-

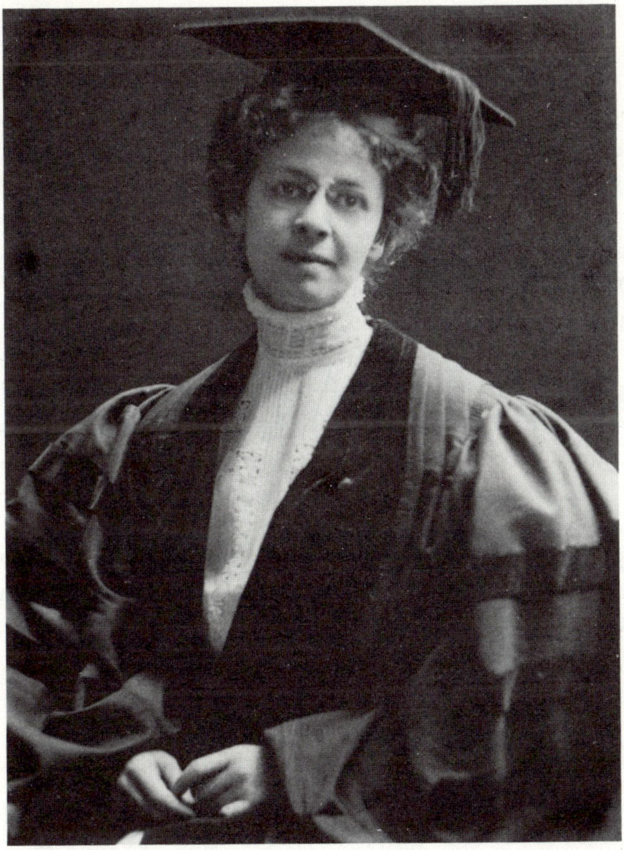

Fig. 3.2 Mary Davies Swartz receives the Ph.D. degree, 1909

tion of Protein Free from Water-Soluble Vitamine" (*Journal of Biological Chemistry*, vol. 39, 1919).

Anton R. Rose became the husband of Mary Swartz following their studies at Yale. Although his major professional interest was in chemistry, he contributed to nutrition through his research in minerals (to be discussed in chapter 5) and also through his interest in the research and writings of his wife and her associates at Teachers College and his continued support of their programs. At the time that Mary Swartz Rose was very active professionally, few women held leadership positions and most husbands of the time did not wish their wives to have careers. Anton Rose wanted his wife to continue her career. He was very cooperative. He claimed that he ate his way through her book *Feeding the Family* because he ate all the foods prepared from the recipes to test them!

Anton Rose's thesis at Yale dealt with phytophosphates: Part 1, A resume of the literature of inosite phosphoric acid with specific reference to its relation to plants; Part 2, The influence of phytin on the growth of lapin seedlings; Part 3, A study of the metabolic and physiologic effects of certain phosphorus compounds with milk cows.

William C. Rose (born 1887) is the only surviving member of the 1908 class at Yale. He is research professor of biochemistry, emeritus, University of Illinois, and lives in New York.

With the discovery and naming of protein in 1839 by Gerardus Mulder, the line of research leading to studies on amino acids began to diverge from that on the components of a complete diet. Until early in the twentieth century, the controversy about protein was with regard to how much protein is necessary for correct nutrition. After the turn of the century, research centered on the different values of pure proteins in animal nutrition.

As late as 1900 only twelve amino acids that are now recognized as components of dietary protein had been discovered, and there was very meager information about them.[22] In 1914 Osborne and Mendel proved that certain amino acids must be included in the food of the growing rat in order to prevent nutritive failure. The work started by Osborne and Mendel stimulated a lifetime of work by William C. Rose. In 1936 he isolated and identified a new amino acid, threonine, which was found to be essential to normal nutrition. From 1942 to 1955 he conducted experiments with human subjects to show that only eight of the ten amino acids that are essential for growth in the rat are essential for the maintenance of nitrogen equilibrium in normal human adults.

Stanley R. Benedict (1884–1936), under Mendel's direction while a student, studied the paths of excretion of several inorganic elements. One year after graduation from Yale, Benedict was appointed to take charge of physiological chemistry at Cornell University College of Medicine in New York City and concentrated on improving analytical methods. He succeeded, through many years of investigations, in devising and perfecting analytical procedures so that chemical analysis became a useful technique for the discovery of the chemical processes in the normal functioning body.[23]

Brief notes on other class members of 1908 follow.

George E. Gage became professor of animal pathology at Massachusetts College and later a physiological chemist with the United States Department of Agriculture. He was concerned with investigations of sodium benzoate.

Warren W. Hilditch, chemist, conducted research in glycosuria, carbohydrate metabolism in relation to complete removal of the thyroid and partial parathyroidectomy, the influence of alcohol in metabolism, acidosis, and the toxicity of organic acids. He went to Syracuse College of Medicine immediately after graduation from Yale and then to positions in clinical laboratories and hospitals in New York City and Newark, New Jersey.

Israel S. Kleiner was in the chemistry department at Tulane University for one year after graduation, and then appointed professor of physiological chemistry at New York Homeopathic Medical College. His research was in experimental diabetes and intermediary metabolism of carbohydrates.

John F. Lyman was professor of agricultural chemistry at Ohio State University. He was interested in animal nutrition and in the metabolism of fats and purines.

Victor C. Myers, physiological chemist, was at Albany Medical College for two years and then became acting director of the laboratories at the Postgraduate Medical School and Hospital, New York. His research interests were in the metabolism of creatine, creatinine, and pyrimidins, pellagra, and blood in health and disease.

Tadasu Saiki became head of the Imperial Institute of Nutrition, Japan.

MARY SWARTZ'S DOCTORAL THESIS

Swartz's doctoral thesis, which was presented to the faculty in 1909, gives an early indication of her lifelong interest in the diets of many persons and her search for comparatively inexpensive food materials that have true nutritive value. Her thesis was entitled "Nutrition Investigations on the Carbohydrates of Lichens, Algae and Related Substances."[24, 25]

Since there had been almost no scientific investigation of the behavior of these substances in the body—although there were special virtues attached to them in the popular mind and even within the medical profession—Swartz decided that their nature and digestibility should be studied. If they were found to have any real nutritive value, a wider use of them could be encouraged since they are widely distributed in nature, are relatively inexpensive, and already form a considerable part of the diet of many persons. If, however, they were found to have no particular value, they should not be relied upon as a source of nutriment in disease (fig. 3.3).

Now, almost seventy years later, Swartz's research is important to us because "dietary fiber" is of great interest due to the large number of serious diseases that have been linked with long-continued intakes of diets low in fiber. Hospitals and clinics and even the general public are using more "high-fiber diets" and "eating more roughage." This is due in many instances to information that is speculative rather than to definitely known and proven facts.

The term "dietary fiber" today is commonly used to refer to components of food known as either cellulose, lignin, or hemicellulose. Cellulose is not attacked by any enzyme of the digestive juices. It is the bulk-inducing component of dietary fiber. Lignin refers to complex indigestible substances that can combine with bile acids to form insoluble substances. That is, cellulose and lignin are indigestible. Hemicelluloses comprise a large group of carbohydrates including mucilages, gums, and pectin. Hemicelluloses can be broken down quite readily by bacteria to form compounds that can be absorbed and yield energy.[26] It was just this last point that Mary Swartz proved in 1909; that is, that the hemicelluloses of algae are utilized by the human body. She found that about 10 to almost 100 percent of their potential calorie value was furnished to the body.

Swartz's method of determining the calorie* value of complex car-

Calories refer to kilocalories throughout the book.

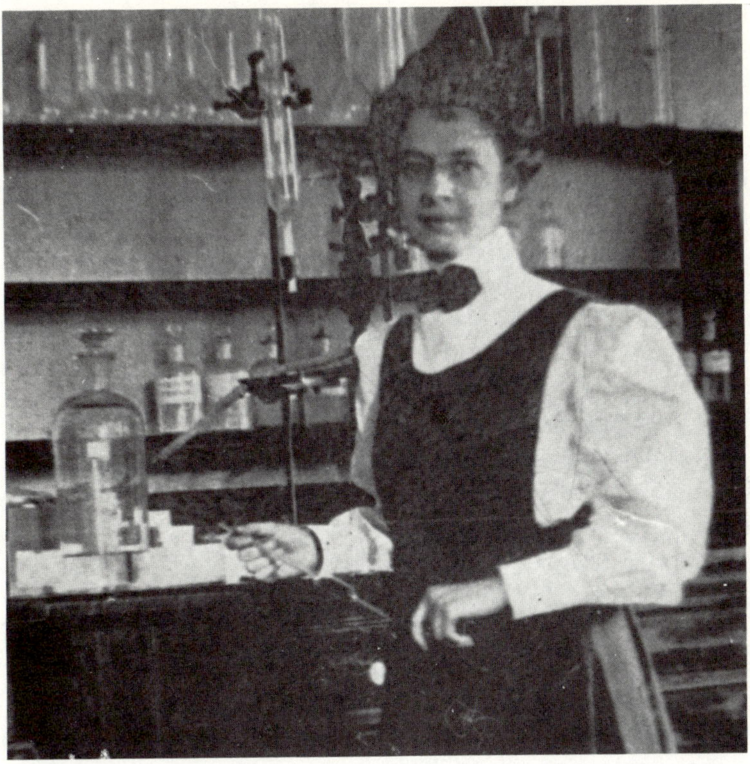

Fig. 3.3 Mary Davies Swartz in the laboratory at Yale University, 1909

bohydrates could be used today, for in the words of Franklin C. Bing:

> Should information about the food value of a substance for human beings be desired, then recourse may be had to human feeding assays, such as Mrs. Rose showed how to perform sixty-five years ago.[27]

A brief review of Swartz's research is in order. She investigated ten species of marine algae, eight of them Hawaiian limu and the other two dulse and Irish moss, knowing that the carbohydrates of algae are chiefly hemicelluloses that are to a great extent water soluble. Most of the carbohydrates were complex in nature, and were grouped with reference to what appeared to be the chief constituent of each. Accordingly, there were five pentosans, eight galactans, two mannans, and two levulins used; except for the levulins, the rest were representative of a large class of materials used by humans for food.

The general method of preparation and the specific procedures used for each of the four types of hemicelluloses will not be described. Bacteriological investigations were carried out because it was reasonable to expect that some hemicelluloses would be attacked and decomposed by bacteria. Therefore, the problem was to find what organisms are most likely to effect decomposition and whether there is an appreciable resultant production of sugar.

It is the physiological investigations that we are especially interested in today. In these experiments, Swartz wished to answer the following questions: (1) To what extent are hemicelluloses digested by animal and vegetable enzymes? (2) Can they be absorbed and utilized without intervention of the alimentary tract? and (3) Do they reappear in the feces? Trials with enzymes, parenteral trials, and feeding experiments were conducted. It is the latter that Bing recommends.

The feeding experiments were carried out with dogs and with healthy, active young women. In the dog experiments, a uniform weight diet of chopped lean meat, lard, and cracker meal was used, and the carbohydrate under investigation was dissolved or suspended in water and mixed with the basal ration. In the human experiments, diets were as uniform as possible with carbohydrates limited almost entirely to bread and crackers made from white flour, potato, and sugar; all cellulose-containing foods such as nuts, fruits, green vegetables, peas and beans, coarse bread and cereals were avoided. The carbohydrates being investigated were added in one of three ways: the gelatinizing carbohydrates were added as blancmange or jelly, the dulse was dissolved in some beverage, and the insoluble preparations were boiled and eaten as a vegetable. Feces were collected and analyzed in both types of experiments.

Swartz's investigations caused her to reiterate Mendel's earlier warning against the assumption that every carbohydrate, by virtue of its chemical composition, is a true nutrient for humans. She found that final conclusions can be drawn only from exact metabolic experiments because the soluble hemicelluloses show great diversity in the digestive tract, some disappearing entirely while others reappear in the feces even up to 100 percent, although they are equally resistant to digestive enzymes in vitro. Lafayette B. Mendel showed his response to her investigations in a letter to Mrs. Rose, dated May 22, 1912 (fig. 3.4).

LAFAYETTE B. MENDEL,
Yale University
NEW HAVEN, CONNECTICUT.

May 22, 1912

My dear Mrs Rose;

I thank you for your kind message of sympathy which I appreciate highly.

The reprints have reached me. I have read your diet-ary study with much interest. It represents a rather novel mode of analysis and one which could be applied in many hospital wards with valuable outcome. Only those who have carefully observed it know how unsatisfactory the diet of the convalescents and other cases not requiring specially ordered food is in many wards.

Professor H. Strauss of Berlin has taken up the inulin problem again, and specifically in the "Therapie der Gegenwart", August 1911. (I can lend you the reprint). We enclose brief series of experiments by Mr. Lewis may interest you in connection with the Salep work.

Your thesis work has been quite widely read and is receiving recognition, as you have doubtless noted.

With greetings to Mr. Rose and you, I am,

Lafayette B. Mendel

Fig. 3.4 Letter to Mary Swartz Rose from Lafayette M. Mendel on her investigations

Subject matter in nutrition is a means to a very definite end—action—MSR

chapter four TEACHERS COLLEGE, COLUMBIA UNIVERSITY

EARLY HISTORY OF TEACHERS COLLEGE

Teachers College was founded in 1887. It grew out of the progressiveness of Grace Hoadley Dodge, the daughter of a wealthy New York merchant, and the foresight of Nicholas Murray Butler, associate professor of philosophy at Columbia College. Along with three or four other young women Miss Dodge had started a philanthropic organization in 1880 called the Kitchen Garden Association as part of the parish work of St. Mark's Church in the Bowery. The purpose of the organization was to help young girls of school age in household economy and thereby assist in improving slum living.[1] Talks to the girls by Miss Dodge on topics such as health, housekeeping, food and marketing, and care of the sick were published in book form by Funk and Wagnalls in 1887. The organization was broadened in 1884 to foster practical education, and was renamed the Industrial Education Association. Although public interest was generated by this action, it was realized that very little could be accomplished without qualified instructors. In 1886 Nicholas Murray Butler became president of the organization. He was imbued with the ideas of President Barnard of Columbia College for a center for the "science and art of education" and pressed for the development of a college for training teachers. He was successful.

The New York College for the Training of Teachers was chartered in 1889 with Butler as its first president. The name was changed to Teachers College in 1892, and the college moved from No. 9 University Place in lower Manhattan to its present site on 120 Street between Broadway and Amsterdam Avenues. In 1893 an agreement was entered into with Columbia and Barnard colleges for reciprocal opportunities and advantages in the granting of degrees. It was not until a little later that the present concept of Columbia University came into being. Then the president of Columbia University became ex-officio the president of Teachers College and the dean of Teachers College became the administrative head of the college. Butler became president of Columbia University in 1901.

James Earl Russell was named the first dean of Teachers College in 1897. He provided the vision and leadership needed at that time. He established four goals for training: general culture, special scholarship, professional knowledge, and technical skill. He believed that the great problem in the training of teachers was knowing how to combine these characteristics in proper proportions.[2] Russell's broad viewpoint enabled him to attract faculty whose work was the keynote for future growth and strength and brought Teachers College to world renown.

Grace Hoadley Dodge had realized the need for teachers who could teach practical education, not only traditional academic subjects. Therefore, in helping to establish Teachers College, she stressed the development of teacher training programs in science as applied to the problems of human beings and everyday living. This aspect of education became a vital part of the developing college. Under Dean Russell the practical courses were grouped in departments such as domestic science, domestic art, and manual training. Helen Kinne, Anna Barrows, Lydia Southard, and May Van Arsdale were some of the early instructors. When Winifred Gibbs became a part-time instructor around 1909, she was effective in relating domestic science to social service in the curriculum. She organized the Home Economics Department of the New York Association for Improving the Condition of the Poor (later the Community Service Society). Even in those early days, there were trained visiting dietitians and/or housekeepers who went to the homes of the poor to assist the mother in better selection and preparation of food and in other household duties.

In 1909 Miss Dodge gave a building in memory of her mother

where Teachers College could provide adequately for the sciences underlying domestic science. This building was named Grace Dodge Hall.

THE NUTRITION PROGRAM AT TEACHERS COLLEGE

It was in 1909 that the nutrition program was established at Teachers College. Henry C. Sherman, professor of food chemistry at Columbia University, had taught a course for Teachers College students since 1904 and held appointments at Teachers College as lecturer in dietetics and dietaries (1906–07) and as professor in 1907. He became the first chairman of the Department of Nutrition and Food Economics in 1909 in the School of Household Arts. Mary Swartz, who returned to Teachers College following graduation at Yale in 1909, was the first full-time staff member in nutrition and received a professorial appointment in 1910. She and Sherman initiated the training program for nutrition teachers, dietitians, and nutritionists.

In the dean's report of 1904, Russell had written "a strong scientific foundation is the prime requisite in all areas of domestic science." He further stated "the Columbia University Department of Applied Chemistry will supplement ours in the chemistry of foods and nutrition by a research course under Professor Henry C. Sherman."

Henry C. Sherman (1875–1955) had received his Ph.D. degree in chemistry at Columbia in 1897 at age twenty-two, then the youngest person to receive the degree at the university. After a year as an assistant in nutrition in the United States Department of Agriculture under Wilbur O. Atwater, Sherman returned to Columbia to specialize in quantitative organic analysis of food products. The intensity of his interest in organic analysis is illustrated by the fact that thirty-six of his first thirty-eight journal papers were of that nature. His interest in enzymes came to light in 1910 with the publication of his first of approximately fifty papers in this field of research, including proof that two of the pure enzymes were proteins.[3] He conducted many early studies in human nutrition, including quantitative studies of total energy; acid-base balance; and iron, calcium, magnesium, phosphorus, protein, and vitamin requirements. His work was notably careful and significant. He insisted that all data be subjected to statistical appraisal, and was one of the first nutrition authors to include this emphasis in his textbook.[4]

Sherman's publications numbered more than three hundred journal papers and a number of books. His textbooks on nutrition soon became the most widely read in their field and his other books were widely accepted. His first text *Methods of Organic Analysis* was published in 1905. He is well known for his second book *Chemistry of Food and Nutrition*, which was published in 1911 and went through eight editions, the last published in 1952, and for *The Nutritional Improvement of Life*, a book that has been called a classic in nutrition.[5] Titles of some of his other books are *Food Products, Food and Health, The Science of Nutrition, Foods: Their Value and Management*, and *Calcium and Phosphorus in Foods and Nutrition*. Sherman's associates, with assistance from the Nutrition Foundation, prepared *Selected Works of Henry Clapp Sherman*, which was published in 1948.

Sherman was dedicated to a cause—the nutritional improvement of life.[6] He was a chemist, nutritionist, teacher, humanitarian, and one of the world's great crusaders.[7] He was a quiet, kindly man. He was one of the founders of the American Institute of Nutrition.

In the autumn of 1909 Mary Swartz gave her first course in dietetics at Teachers College. There were seventeen women in her first class. All nutrition classes were held in Room 401 in Dodge Hall, a combination classroom and laboratory that she had planned and equipped. She believed:

> It is essential that laboratory practice with actual food materials accompany instruction in the quantitative aspects of dietetics, and it is advantageous even in considering the qualitative side to present a dietary in concrete form. A place must therefore be provided where weighing and measuring of food materials and cooking and serving of days' rations for individuals and groups can be done by a whole class.[8]

Her office was also on the fourth floor of Dodge Hall (fig. 4.1). There was a nutrition research laboratory and a small animal laboratory on the fifth floor. Adjoining the laboratory was a suite of small rooms (kitchen, dining room, bedroom, bath, and living room) originally planned as a practice apartment for home economics students, but later used by nutrition research students while carrying out human investigations.

The Teachers College catalog began listing courses offered in nutrition in 1903. Tables 4.1 and 4.2 indicate the offerings in the early days of the nutrition program.

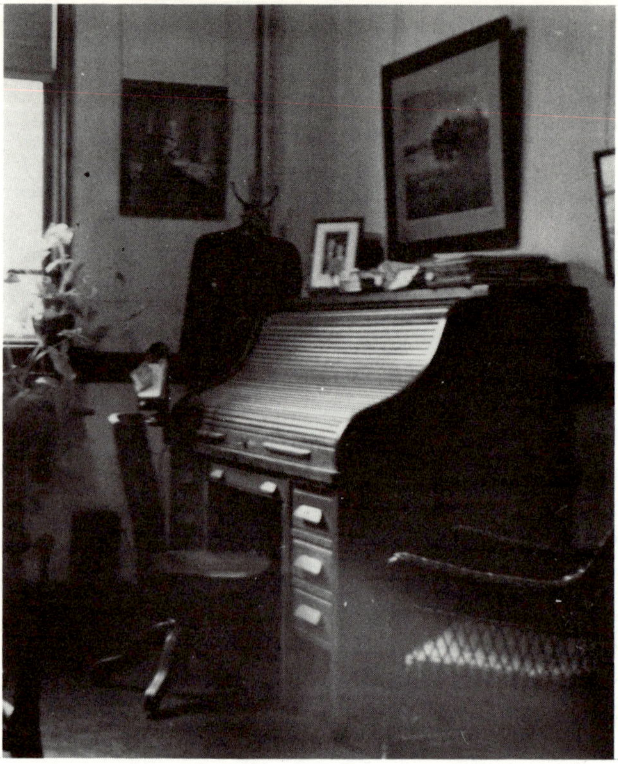

Fig. 4.1 Mary Swartz Rose's desk in Room 408 Dodge Hall, Teachers College

The names of professorial and instructional staff in the nutrition program are given in table 4.3 (persons in the preliminary period are given in table 4.1). Sherman taught a number of courses with Rose until 1924 when Grace MacLeod became a full-time assistant professor. Sherman continued to participate in the nutrition seminars for many years. Mary Swartz Rose was promoted from assistant professor to associate professor in 1918 and then to professor of nutrition in 1923.

Grace MacLeod (1878–1962) had taken her B.S. degree in chemistry at the Massachusetts Institute of Technology in 1901. She had been a student of Ellen H. Richards, an early lecturer who taught sanitary chemistry, who was instrumental in establishing the American Home Economics Association, serving as its first president. Grace MacLeod had taught at the Mt. Hermon School for Boys and at Technical High

TABLE 4.1 Courses Offered through the Teachers College Food and Nutrition Program, 1903–10[9]

Year	*Course*	*Teacher*
1903–14	Foods	Miss Mary Vail, Miss Helen Day
	Foods, Advanced Course	Prof. Helen Kinne, Miss Vail, Miss Day
Summer 1904	Chemistry of Food and Nutrition	Dr. Henry C. Sherman
1904–05	Foods	Miss Vail, Miss Day
	Foods, Advanced Course	Prof. Kinne, Miss Vail, Miss Day
Summer 1905	Chemistry of Nutrition	Dr. Sherman
	Proximate Organic and Sanitary Analysis	Dr. Sherman
1905–06	Foods	Miss Vail, Miss Day
	Foods, Advanced Course	Prof. Kinne, Miss Vail, Miss Day
Summer 1906	Proximate Organic and Sanitary Analysis	Prof. Sherman
	Chemistry of Nutrition	Prof. Sherman
	Foods	Miss Eliza Benton
1906–07	Dietaries, Nutritive Values and Costs	Prof. Sherman, Mrs. Ellen Richards, and special lecturers
Summer 1907	Elementary Physiological Chemistry	Prof. Sherman
	Chemistry of Nutrition	Prof. Sherman
	Proximate Organic and Sanitary Analysis	Prof. Sherman, Mr. Sinclair
	Foods	Miss Benton
1907–08	Dietaries, Nutritive Values and Costs—1st half year	Prof. Sherman and assistant
	—2nd half year	Prof. Mary Nutting, Mrs. Richards, and special lecturers
	Food and Dietaries	Miss Benton
	Metabolism and Dietetics	Prof. Sherman
Summer 1908	Elementary Physiological Chemistry	Prof. Sherman
	Chemistry of Nutrition	Prof. Sherman
	Organic and Sanitary Analysis	Prof. Sherman and assistant
	Foods	Miss Benton, Miss Wilson

TABLE 4.1—*Continued*

Year	*Course*	*Teacher*
	Research under Prof. Sherman	
1908–09	Dietaries, Nutritive Values and Costs—1st half year	Prof. Sherman and assistant
	—2nd half year	Prof. Nutting, Mrs. Richards, and special lecturers
	Food and Dietaries	(not listed)
	Metabolism and Dietetics	Prof. Sherman
Summer 1909	Chemistry of Nutrition	Prof. Sherman
	Organic and Sanitary Analysis	Prof. Sherman
	Food Analysis and Inspection	Prof. Sherman
	Foods	Miss Benton, Miss Wilson
	Research under Prof. Sherman	
1909–10	Dietetics	Prof. Mary Swartz
	Nutrition	Prof. Sherman
	Nutrition and Dietetics	Prof. Sherman and assistant
	Practicum in Nutrition	Prof. Sherman
Summer 1910	Dietetics	Prof. Mary Swartz
	Institutional Dietaries	Miss Corbett
	Nutrition (same as Chemistry of Nutrition)	Prof. Sherman

TABLE 4.2 Summary of Nutrition Courses, 1910–40

Nutrition Laboratory Methods

Investigations of the nutritive value of foods; feeding and metabolism studies; dietary studies and interpretations

Professor Sherman, 1910–11

Professor Rose and others, 1911–19

1919—name changed to Introduction to Laboratory Research

Practicum in Nutrition and Food Economics

Introduces graduate students to investigation of problems in nutrition and food economics

Professor Sherman, 1910–11

Professors Sherman and Rose, 1911–19

1919—name changed to Progress in Nutrition

Table 4.2—*Continued*

Nutrition
Reviews nutritive functions and fuel values of food.
Professor Sherman, 1910–12
Professors Sherman and Rose, 1912–19

Dietetics
Fundamental principles of human nutrition applied to feeding individuals, families, and larger groups under varying physiological, economic, and social conditions
Professor Swartz, 1910–11
Professor Rose, 1911–14
Professor Rose and others, 1914–19

Institutional Dietetics
Administrative duties of dietitians; practical problems of food supplies under normal and abnormal conditions
Miss Corbett, 1910–12

Elementary Food Economics
Nontechnical discussions of functions and nutritive value of foods; the feeding of families and larger groups
Professors Sherman and Swartz, 1910–11
Professors Sherman and Rose, 1911–13
Professor Sherman and others, 1914–18

Investigation in Nutrition and Food Economics
Qualified students conduct investigation under individual direction
Professors Sherman and Rose, 1911–19

Dietetics of Childhood
Professor Rose and Miss McCormick, 1911–12

Food and Nutrition
Broad survey of nutritive values of food and nutrition requirements of the body; for non-majors
Professor Rose, 1912–14
Miss McCormick and Miss Field, 1914–18
1919—name changed to *Nutrition and Health*

In 1919 the courses Feeding the Sick and Fieldwork in Dietetics were added to the offerings.

In 1921 the course Feeding the Sick was expanded to one in Nutrition in Disease, and Fieldwork in Metabolism was introduced. In 1924 a course in Problems in Energy Metabolism was added. A course called Advanced Nutrition surveying nutrition needs throughout the human life cycle was introduced in 1927, about the same time that Research Problems in Teaching Nutrition was formally established. A doctoral Seminar in Nutrition was added in 1932 and Readings in Nutrition in 1935.

TABLE 4.3 Staff of the Nutrition Program to 1975

	*Professorial Staff**	*Instructional Staff**
1889–1908		
Preliminary period	(see table 4.1)	(see table 4.1)
1909–40		
Dr. Henry C. Sherman first chairman 1909 Dr. Mary Swartz Rose full time 1909–40 in charge 1910–40	Dr. Grace MacLeod 1924–40 Dr. Clara Mae Taylor 1939–40	Mary McCormick 1911–18 Ada Field 1914–18 Harriet Barto 1918–21 Grace MacLeod 1919–24 Emma Winslow 1920–22 Margaret Sandels 1921–22 Margaret Hessler (Brooks) 1924–26 Hazel Stiebeling 1924–26 Clara Mae Taylor 1926–39 Elda Robb 1927–29 and 1932–33 Adeline Missal 1929–32
1940–44		
Dr. Grace MacLeod in charge	Dr. Grace MacLeod 1940–44 Dr. Clara Mae Taylor 1940–44	Orrea F. Pye 1940–42 Edna Sostman 1943–44 Mary Bal
1944–63		
Dr. Clara Mae Taylor in charge	Dr. Clara Mae Taylor 1944–63 Dr. Orrea F. Pye 1944–63 Dr. Bertlyn Bosley 1st semester 1944 Robert Goodhart, M.D. (Lecturer) 1950–53	Edna Sostman 1944–53 Dr. Anne Caldwell 1944–48 Dorothy Williams 1946–48 Lorraine Gates 1947–50 Juanita Archibald 1947–50 Nelle Sailor 1950–60

TABLE 4.3—*Continued*

	*Professorial Staff**	*Instructional Staff**
1963–75 Dr. Orrea F. Pye in charge 1963–72 Dr. Mary McCann in charge 1972–73 Dr. Orrea F. Pye acting chairman 1973–75	Dr. Orrea F. Pye 1963–75 Dr. Eleanor Williams 1966–72 Dr. Bertlyn Bosley (Adjunct) Dr. Juanita Eagles (Adjunct) **Dr. Mary Dumm 1970– Dr. Mary Bal (Lecturer) Dr. Edna Sostman (Lecturer) 1963–64 George Christakis, M.D. (Lecturer) 1970–73 Roy Brown, M.D. (Lecturer) 1972–73 Mary McCann, M.D. 1972–73	Marion Abbot 1964–65 Rose Mirenda 1964–65 Claire Brooks 1964–66 Marion Mike 1965–70 Carol Fritz 1969–71 Luise Light 1969–73 Rachel Lipsky 1970–72 Reva Frankle 1970–75 **Joan Gussow 1971–75 Ruth Eshleman 1972–73 **Marilyn Hesser 1972– **Katherine McCloy 1972–

**Plus Teaching Assistants*
***Staff who continued after 1975, under Professor Joan Gussow*

School, both in Massachusetts, from 1901 to 1910. Then she was appointed instructor in chemistry and physics at Pratt Institute, New York, and began taking courses at Columbia University. Her first course, the Nutrition Seminar conducted by Professors Sherman and Rose, was the inspiration for her lifetime interest in nutrition as a science. She was able as a student to make a real contribution to the seminar because much of the literature in chemistry and nutrition at that time was published in German, in which she had an excellent background. She received her master's degree from Columbia in 1914. From 1917 to 1919 she was employed as assistant editor of the *Journal of Industrial and Engineering Chemistry*. She returned to Teachers College as an instructor in nutrition in 1919 and received the Ph.D. degree from Columbia in 1924 working under Mary Swartz Rose. Her promotion to professorship at Teachers College was wait-

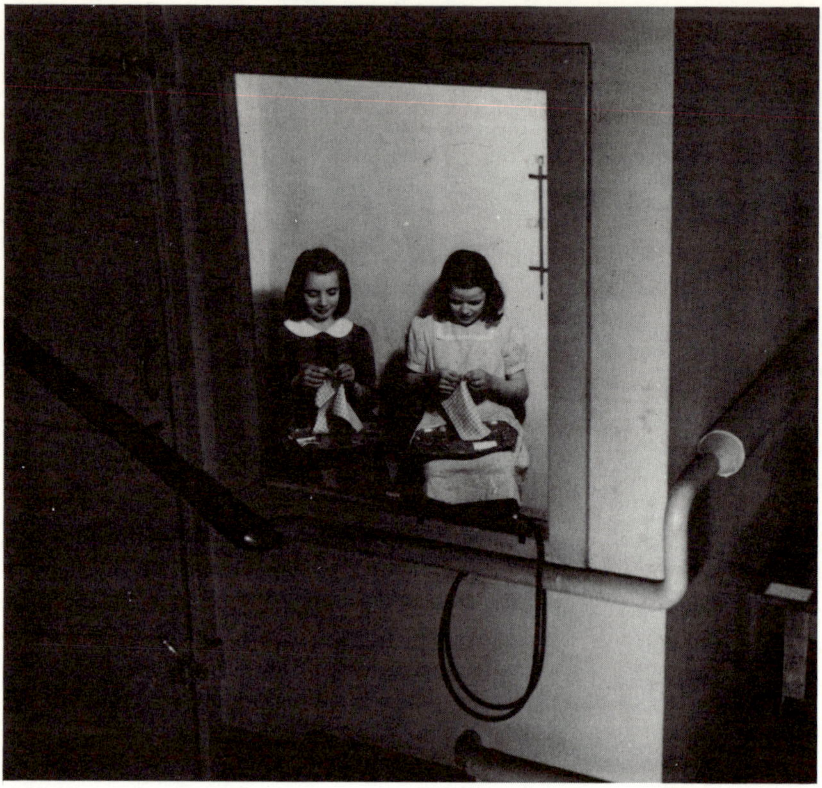

Fig. 4.2 Using the respiration chamber at Teachers College to measure the energy expenditure of sewing

ing on her desk when she returned from commencement exercises at which her doctoral degree had been conferred.[10]

MacLeod was a dedicated and tireless research worker who supervised the animal laboratory, ordering supplies, checking equipment, and always making sure that the basic essentials for research were in prime condition. Her most active field of research was in energy metabolism. Her doctoral dissertation, "Studies of the Normal Basal Energy Requirement," initiated many investigations carried out in the nutrition laboratory at Teachers College. She superintended the setting up of the respiration chamber in the Child Development Institute and again when it was moved to the college (fig. 4.2). She was responsible for acquiring other equipment for energy metabolism studies and for its installation. MacLeod and Rose organized their research activities well, each having her role in dissertation research. MacLeod supervised several Ph.D. dissertations dealing with energy metabolism (see table 5.2—Potgieter, Robb, Williams, Taylor, Thompson). After Rose's retirement, MacLeod directed the following dissertation investigations:

1942 Robertson, Mary E. "A Study of the Energy Metabolism and Mechanical Efficiency of Children Six to Eight Years of Age"

1942 Lamb, Mina Wolf "A Comparison of Energy Expenditure of Boys and Young Men"

1942 Houghton, Dorothy "The Utilization of Iron from Foods Studied by Two Methods"

1943 Pye, Orrea F. "The Utilization of Iron from Different Foods by Normal Young Rats"

1944 Caldwell, Anne B. "The Effect of Age and Diet on the Storage of (1) Vitamin A in Liver and (2) Riboflavin in Liver and Muscle in the Albino Rat"

1944 Bosley, Bertlyn "The Effects of Change from a Poor to a Good Diet Measured by Growth, Calcium Storage, and Hemoglobin Levels"

1944 Langwill, Katheryn E. "The Effect of Anoxia on the Ascorbic Acid, pH, and Titratable Acidity of the Urine of Rats Fed Various Diets"

1945 Phillips, Margaret L. "The Effect of Diets of Different Iron Content on Hemoglobin Values of Rats during Pregnancy and Lactation"

From 1922 to 1928 MacLeod was a cooperating investigator in energy metabolism with the Nutrition Laboratory of the Carnegie Institution, Boston, and published three articles with the director, F. G. Benedict.

During World War II, MacLeod was chairman of the Food and Nutrition Council of Greater New York, an organization she had helped to establish in the twenties. She also served as chairman of the Nutrition Committee of the Greater New York Area, serving on the National Nutrition Program of the War Food Administration. She was chairman of the Nutrition Advisory Board, New York Chapter of the American Red Cross; member of the Advisory Committee of the East Harlem Health Center; member of the Executive Committee of the

New York City Food and Nutrition Program and cochairman of the Planning Committee; member of the Nutrition Advisory Committee of the Henry Street Visiting Nurse Service; and member of the Advisory Board of the Interstate Dairy Council of Philadelphia. She was active in many professional organizations. She was an associate editor of the *Journal of Nutrition,* 1936–39, and continued to serve on its editorial board, 1940–45. She served as a member of the editorial board of the *Journal of the American Dietetic Association,* 1940–44.[11]

Her students had great appreciation of Grace MacLeod's teaching abilities. Although demanding meticulous performance in laboratory and classroom, she was gracious and patient in assisting the student. Her strong convictions, sincerity, and outspoken manner of speaking brought respect and admiration from students and associates. She had a special talent for writing concise reviews and editorial assessments of research studies.

Mary Swartz Rose and Grace MacLeod, devoted friends and associates, established a strong program for training students in nutrition. These two, with different backgrounds and personalities, complemented each other in many ways and worked together in a common effort to provide the best possible training for the students.[12]

Grace MacLeod directed the nutrition program following Rose's retirement in 1940. When she retired in 1944, nutrition students and friends honored her by establishing the Grace MacLeod Scholarship Fund.

One cannot tell the story of Mary Swartz Rose and the development of the nutrition program at Teachers College without writing of her coworkers Henry C. Sherman and Grace MacLeod. The primary author, Juanita Archibald Eagles, also wishes to call attention to the roles played by the coauthors of this biography. Both were students of Mary Swartz Rose. Clara Mae Taylor was an associate of Rose for many years. Orrea F. Pye worked with Rose while a graduate student. Each in turn was in charge of the nutrition program at Teachers College. Both continued in the tradition of Mary Swartz Rose, adapting positively to new developments in the science of nutrition and the needs of nutrition educators.

Clara Mae Taylor came to Teachers College as a student in 1916, working toward the B.S. degree that she received in 1920. She then taught in a junior high school in Bridgeton, New Jersey (1920–22), and was an instructor in home economics at Rhode Island State College

(1922–26). She received the A.M. degree in education at Teachers College in 1923.

Mary Swartz Rose called Taylor back to Teachers College in 1926, first as an assistant in nutrition for one semester and then as an instructor, thus providing Taylor an opportunity to work toward her Ph.D. degree, which she received in 1937. As Taylor stated in "Reminiscences of Mary Swartz Rose," "The Rose, MacLeod and Taylor team worked harmoniously together with one goal in mind—that of promoting a strong training program in nutrition. Nothing was too great a task if we were convinced that it was for the good of our students."[13] Taylor became an assistant professor in 1939, an associate professor in 1943, and a full professor in 1948. Taylor assumed the leadership of the nutrition program following MacLeod's retirement in 1944.

In 1944 Taylor obtained a grant from the U.S. Department of Agriculture to study the energy expenditure of children. Professor Emeritus MacLeod served as a consultant on the research project for several years. The U.S. Department of Agriculture supported this project for twelve years and also another research project to study the energy expenditures of younger and older women for a period of four years. These research activities not only served to increase the nutrition teaching staff but also provided research experience and financial assistance for students working toward advanced degrees. Seventeen students working on the energy studies held staff appointments and many others assisted on an hourly basis.

Taylor served on the staffs of the Horace Mann Lincoln Institute of School Experimentation (1943–46) and of several educational surveys. She directed a nutrition education project supported by General Mills (1947–53). This project made it possible for Taylor to establish special nutrition education programs at Teachers College leading to (1) a Professional Diploma requiring two years of graduate study and (2) a Doctor of Education degree in nutrition education. The Ed.D. degree in nutrition education was the first of its kind in the United States (awarded first to Juanita Archibald [Eagles] in 1952). Practical experience for students was obtained by working directly with classroom teachers, children, and parents in public and private schools in the university area. A second grant in nutrition education provided by Morningside Heights, Inc. made it possible to continue the program (1955–57). The enthusiasm generated stimulated an interest in nutrition education programs in a number of schools in the Greater New York area. These programs were continued under the direction of Taylor until she retired. The Ed.D. degree enabled the prospective nutrition educator to select from the many courses in educational psychology, sociology, and other social and behavioral sciences offered at Teachers College that are so important to leadership roles in nutrition education. The special project required for the completion of the degree could be selected from the multiple problems in nutrition education facing the school and community.

Taylor directed a research project with funds from the Florida Citrus Commission to study the effect of different levels of ascorbic acid in the life of guinea pigs on health, reproduction, and survival (1954–59).

Mary Swartz Rose often stressed the importance of continuing research when talking with Clara Mae Taylor about the future of the nutrition program. It enriched the teaching program and helped insure the continuation of the training program during periods of reorganization.

Taylor established a course in 1945 dealing with Nutrition and Community Health for teachers, public health workers, and nutritionists. In 1946, under her direction, an orientation course in Nutrition in Social Work and Public Health was introduced; in 1947 she initiated a formal program in public health nutrition to meet the requirements of the federal Children's Bureau and the national Association of Directors of Graduate Programs in Public Health Nutrition. The new training program included courses offered by other schools of Columbia University, the School of Public Health, and the School of Social Work, and at a later date, the Institute of Nutrition Sciences. The program included concomitant field experience in health and welfare agencies in New York City and a block of two months internship in a department of public health. When the orientation course for majors was established, a course for non-majors replaced Nutrition and Community Health and was called Nutrition Education in School and Community.

In the 1960s, the course in advanced nutrition was expanded. The orientation course in public health nutrition was refocused as Nutrition in Community Programs. A course in Fieldwork and Observations of Nutrition Programs was identified as different from the course in Fieldwork in Nutrition and Public Health.

Taylor retired in 1963. Her students and colleagues established the Clara Mae Taylor Fellowship Fund as a tribute to her thirty-seven years of service to the nutrition program at Teachers College.

Orrea Florence Pye came to Teachers College as a doctoral student for the academic year 1935–36. She had obtained a B.S. degree in chemistry from Douglass College in 1931 and an M.S. degree in nutrition from Syracuse University in 1934. At Mary Swartz Rose's suggestion that it would be desirable to gain more experience before completing the doctoral degree, she accepted a temporary position as junior food economist in the U.S. Department of Agriculture working directly under Hazel K. Stiebeling. In 1938 Pye accepted an assistant professorship at the University of Alabama, where she was responsible for initiating a program in nutrition. With summers free to study, she continued with the doctoral program at Teachers College, and in 1940 returned full time to complete the requirements for the Ph.D. degree in nutrition. In 1942 she accepted a professorship in nutrition at the Woman's College of the University of North Carolina.

In 1944 Pye returned to Teachers College, first as visiting professor, then as associate professor working part-time as a nutrition chemist under the U.S. Department of Agriculture grant for studies of energy requirements. In 1959 she became a full professor. From the time of Grace MacLeod's retirement in 1944, Pye had been associated with Taylor in the development of the nutrition program at Teachers College.

Upon Taylor's retirement in 1963, Pye assumed leadership of the nutrition program. Two new courses were introduced. One was The Behavioral Aspects of the Nutritionist's Role. Sociologists, psychologists, and/or anthropologists joined the seminars from time to time to help nutrition students in recognizing and dealing with psychosocial problems encountered in working with clients in clinics and community activities. The other was a course developed by Instructor Joan Gussow called Nutritional Ecology.

A new degree course of study was introduced by Pye, the Master of Education, a two-year program that included a special thesis project. This program enabled students who had already obtained a one-year master's degree to take special courses required in public health nutrition or to expand studies into a specialty such as maternal and child health, gerontology, or clinical nutrition.

Because of a change in policy of the federal government, an overall grant for public health nutrition training was given directly to the college rather than individually to students. This policy made possible a larger number of full-time majors in public health nutrition at Teachers College, including those working on M.Ed. and Ed.D. levels. It also necessitated changes in placement practices for supervised field training. Orrea F. Pye developed a liaison with the Nutrition Division of the Community Medicine Department of Mount Sinai School of Medicine. This arrangement enabled Teachers College nutrition and public health majors to work in medical teams in the East Harlem community and to work in the Mount Sinai Medical School Apprentice Program in the summers. These changes were in line with new directives for public health nutrition field training approved by the Association of Graduate Programs in Public Health Nutrition. Other Teachers College nutrition students had supervised field experiences in states or other countries as previously was the custom.

Pye also initiated Public Health Institutes during the summer sessions permitting continuing education credit for nutritionists and dietitians.

In September 1972 Pye became professor emeritus of nutrition. Mary McCann, M.D., who had come to Teachers College for the previous spring term, assumed the responsibility of directing the nutrition program. McCann left in the spring of 1973, and Pye returned as acting chairman that autumn.

In 1974 a conference was held at Teachers College in honor of the 65th year of the nutrition program. It was called "Education in Nutrition—Looking Forward from the Past."

In March 1975 the "Orrea F. Pye Symposium" was held at Teachers College to honor Pye, which dealt with the nutrition educator's response to world hunger. In September 1975 Pye retired as acting head of the program, but held the title of research associate in nutrition until 1977.

The nutrition program at Teachers College, developed under the leadership of Henry C. Sherman, Mary Swartz Rose, Grace MacLeod, Clara Mae Taylor, and Orrea F. Pye (fig. 4.3), began in the School of Household Arts early in the present century, transferred to the Department of Science Education in the mid-1950s, and in 1968 became one of the program areas in the new Division of Health Services, Sciences and Education. It was called the Nutrition Program and administered under the division directly, which was equivalent to departmental status, from 1968 on.

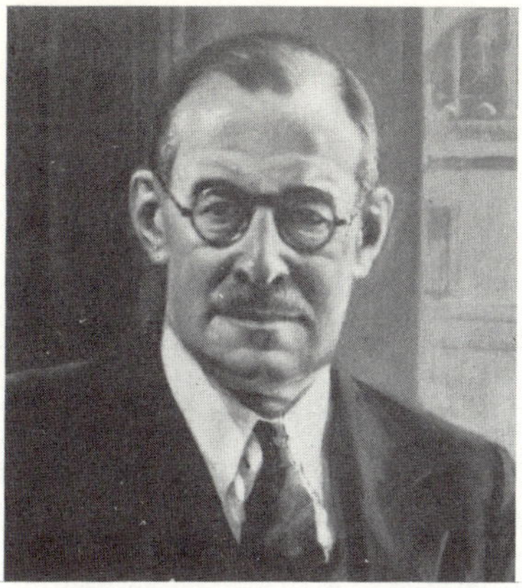

Henry C. Sherman

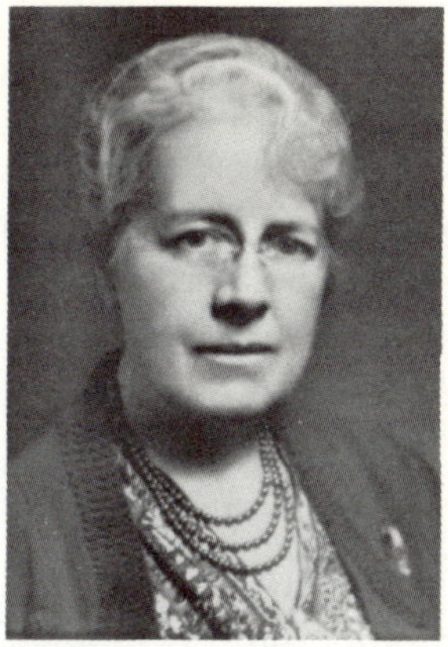

Grace MacLeod

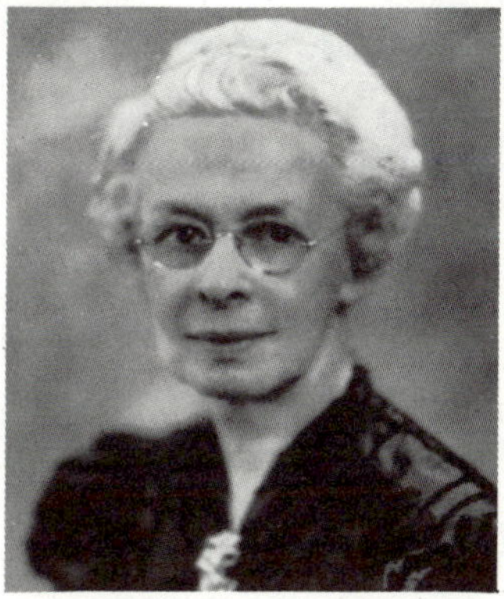

Mary Swartz Rose

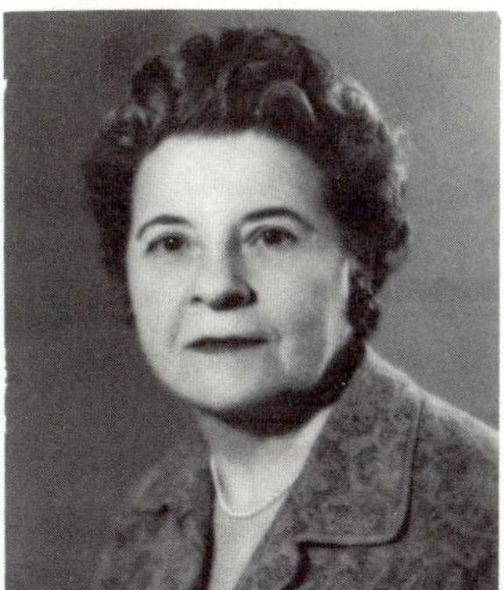

Clara Mae Taylor

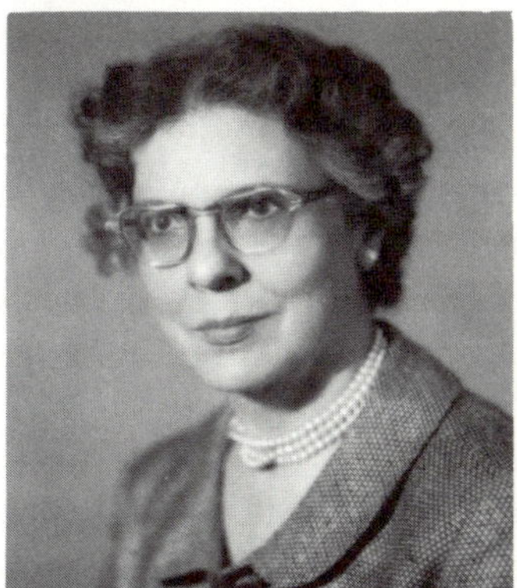

Orrea F. Pye

Fig. 4.3 Leaders of the nutrition program at Teachers College, 1909–74

Dr. Joan Gussow became chairperson of the Program in Nutrition in September 1975.

INSTRUCTIONAL MATERIALS USED BY MARY SWARTZ ROSE

It is interesting to note that the words "nutrition" and "dietetics" were used early in the century to indicate one field of study. Mary Swartz Rose, however, from the very beginning differentiated between nutrition and dietetics. She included her definitions of these two words in an article entitled, "University Teaching of Nutrition and Dietetics in the United States" (1935), the first time that separate and different meanings for the terms appeared in print. Rose stated:

> Nutrition deals with the scientific laws governing the requirements of human beings for maintenance, growth, activity, reproduction and lactation; dietetics with their practical application to individuals or groups, in health and also in sickness.[14]

In 1909 Teachers College offered training in nutrition and in dietetics along with training in principles of education, an unusual opportunity in a school. It also offered study in physiological chemistry as a prerequisite to the study of advanced nutrition, the first school to do so. Many teachers from other schools came to Teachers College to take both physiological chemistry and nutrition courses.

Rose found that she needed information not available in published form for her classes. A list of books used for reference purposes in nutrition courses at Teachers College, annotations by Sherman and Rose,[15] is given in Appendix A, page 162. There was no satisfactory textbook in nutrition until 1911 when Sherman's *Chemistry of Food and Nutrition* was published. The purpose of the book was to present the principles of the chemistry of foods and nutrition with special reference to the food requirements of humans and to also present the criteria that should underlie judgment of the nutritive value and economy of foods. The major portion of the book dealt with organic foodstuffs, their metabolism, and their requirements by the body. Sherman pointed out, however, that it is not safe to assume that mineral elements will be present in sufficient quantities just because carbohydrates, fats, and proteins are supplied in required amounts by the diet. He believed that compounds of iron may be regarded in many ways as connecting links between organic and inorganic (mineral) foodstuffs and body constituents because of their prominence in general metabolism and in activities of specialized cells.[16] He emphasized the need for quantitative investigations of the mineral content of foods and of their requirements in human nutrition, particularly of iron, calcium, and phosphorus. In fact, these investigations were started early in the present century chiefly by the cooperation of Columbia University and the U.S. Department of Agriculture and by the New York Association for Improving the Condition of the Poor (now Community Service Society). Recognition of the importance of the mineral elements in nutrition was one of the features that marked the twentieth century as the era of the newer knowledge of nutrition.[17]

With *Chemistry of Foods and Nutrition* providing a reliable and scholarly text for the nutrition courses, Rose began work on materials for the student of dietetics. She realized the importance of the quantitative study of foods. Since most of the available information on food values was expressed as percentage composition, in practical use the student wasted a great deal of time on tedious calculations, time better spent in the comparative study of food values. Accordingly, Rose developed tables giving food values for (1) 100-calorie portions, a convenient unit for planning a day's food intake to yield a definite number of calories; (2) the gram, the unit of weight for scientific workers; (3) the ounce, the common unit for small families; and (4) the pound, the unit for large families and institutions. These tables were included in Rose's *A Laboratory Handbook for Dietetics* published in 1912, the result of meticulous laboratory weighing of foods in many forms by Rose and students working under her direction.

Along with the tables, *A Laboratory Handbook for Dietetics* also included a series of problems in dietary calculations, worked out step by step, since the student of dietetics must know the processes for calculation even though labor-saving tables and devices are encouraged. Brief statements of conditions affecting food requirements, with appropriate data, were included.[18] Rose revised the *Handbook* three times; Clara Mae Taylor and Grace MacLeod prepared the fifth edition as *Rose's Laboratory Handbook for Dietetics* in 1949.

In the 1920s Rose developed an abbreviated method of expressing relative nutritive values of foods in shares. A "share" of any dietary essential was one-thirtieth of the day's requirement. The new simplified method of denoting food values in shares was used in the book by Rose entitled *Foundations of Nutrition* published in 1927.[19] Two of Rose's former students and staff members cooperated in the development of the method: Margaret C. Hessler first suggested the use of the word "share" and Hazel K. Stiebeling prepared the share table for the appendix of the book. The share system was a popular one and made possible graphic presentation. Dietary evaluation by this system was based on key major nutrients occuring naturally in foods. The same foods could be depended on as sources of other major and minor, and possibly unknown, nutrients. The share system remained valid until the widespread use of highly processed foods irregularly fortified with some nutrients occurred in recent years.

Foundations of Nutrition was intended for beginning college students who wanted some understanding of the significance of food in their own lives and the significance of nutrition to health. Fundamental principles of human nutrition were presented in terms that called for no highly specialized training in the natural sciences. Each essential factor in an adequate diet was discussed with some reference to its historical development, with many references to animal experimentation and with an indication of the food sources of the particular dietary essential. Included as factors were sources of energy; body-building materials; the minerals phosphorus, calcium, iron, iodine, sulfur, sodium, chlorine, potassium, and magnesium; and the vitamins A, B, C, D, and E. An interesting analogy between building a diet and building a house was made in the chapter "Contributions of an Adequate Diet." Rose portrayed foods as resembling wall, door, window, and other units that are purchased already built to be fitted together. Foods are the units one buys; one does not buy calories, protein, minerals, etc. Foods are assembled for a diet, the building units for a house. In 1920 Anton and Mary Rose had begun to build such a house—their beautiful home in Edgewater—by selecting already built units to be assembled to make the type of house they desired.

Graham Lusk's letter expresses Rose's contribution through her book *Foundations of Nutrition* (fig. 4.4).

Mary Swartz Rose revised *Foundations of Nutrition* twice. *Foundations of Nutrition* and *A Laboratory Handbook for Dietetics* had become a vital part of all home economics teaching. The third edition of *Foundations* was in use in more than three hundred fifty institutions. One or

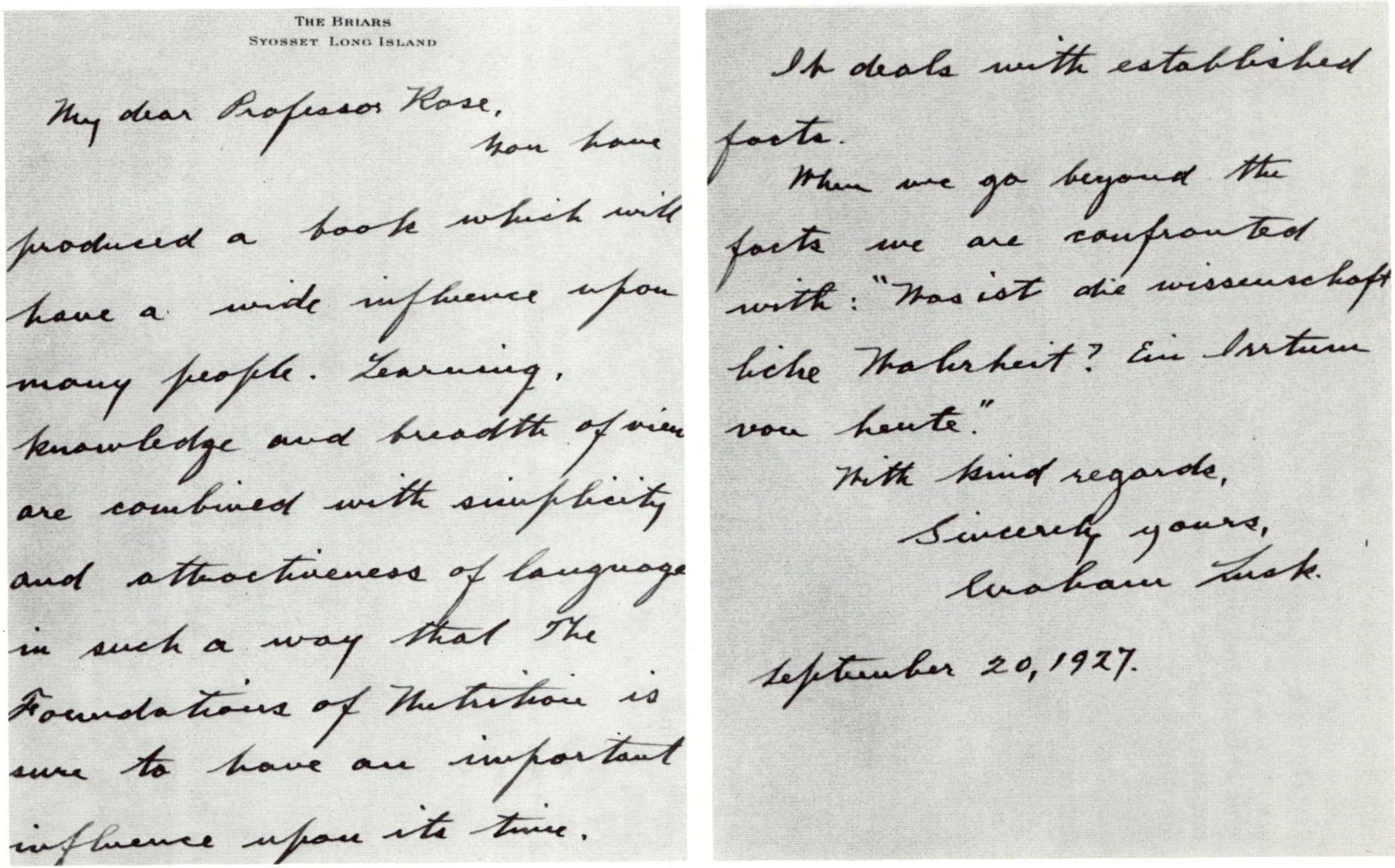

THE BRIARS
SYOSSET LONG ISLAND

My dear Professor Rose,

You have produced a book which will have a wide influence upon many people. Learning, knowledge and breadth of view are combined with simplicity and attractiveness of language in such a way that The Foundations of Nutrition is sure to have an important influence upon its time.

It deals with established facts.

When we go beyond the facts we are confronted with: "Was ist die wissenschaftliche Wahrheit? Ein Irrtum von heute."

With kind regards,

Sincerely yours,

Graham Lusk.

September 20, 1927.

Fig. 4.4 Letter to Mary Swartz Rose from Graham Lusk on the publication of Rose's book, Foundations of Nutrition

both of these books had been adopted by forty-three state colleges and universities.[20] The *Journal of the American Medical Association* stated that *Foundations of Nutrition* should be in the library of every person interested in foods and nutrition. *The American Consumer* recommended it to every consumer and consumer group interested in obtaining the best health results from diet. A fourth edition (1944) entitled *Rose's Foundations of Nutrition* was written by Grace MacLeod and Clara Mae Taylor. A fifth edition (1956) by Clara Mae Taylor and Grace MacLeod and a sixth edition (1966) by Clara Mae Taylor and Orrea F. Pye, both called *Foundations of Nutrition,* were published.

Tables of food values using the share unit were published in *Food Values of Recipes in Shares and Vitamin Units* by Mary Swartz Rose and Clara Mae Taylor in 1931 and revised in 1936.[21] Taylor extensively revised and enlarged the original material, publishing it as *Food Values in Shares and Weights* in 1942 and then again in 1959.[22]

It is research that keeps one's mind alive—MSR

chapter five ROSE'S RESEARCH CONTRIBUTIONS

SCOPE OF RESEARCH INTERESTS

The years 1909 to 1940 when Mary Swartz Rose was active at Teachers College witnessed tremendous advances in knowledge through research in the four major areas of nutrition: energy, proteins and amino acids, minerals, and vitamins.

Thus, Rose received her doctoral training at a propitious time, and she made important contributions in each of these areas.[1]

Because she had worked under Mendel, Rose was well acquainted with the most dependable research methods of the day. She continued to keep abreast of new developments as a member of the prestigious research group, the American Society for Biological Chemists, founded in 1906. In 1928 she was one of the founders of the American Institute of Nutrition when, as she stated, there was a need for a closer organization of nutrition investigators because of the great volume of specialized research in nutrition.[2] Close liaison to Sherman's Department of Chemistry at Columbia also made the supportive setting of Teachers College very favorable for research.

She advanced knowledge of many types of food. She carried on extensive research in nutrition education and developed the importance of nutrition as a subject of instruction from the grade school to the university. The nutrition of children was one of her major interests. She became the great interpreter of laboratory findings, and their value took on importance as practical applications were made to the daily lives of people.[3] The titles of some of her published researches (table 5.1) show the breadth and symmetry of the development of her research in nutrition, some of which she conducted independently and some in collaboration with others.

TABLE 5.1 Titles of Researches (Exclusive of Nutrition Education), with Date of Publication

"Nutrition Investigations on the Carbohydrates of Lichens, Algae and Related Substances," 1911

"A Dietary Study in a Children's Hospital," 1912

"The Biological Efficiency of Potato Nitrogen," 1917

"Creatinuria in Women," 1917

"Calcium Requirement of Maintenance in Man," 1920

"Some Human Digestion Experiments with Raw White of Egg," 1920

"Experiments on the Utilization of the Calcium of Carrots by Man," 1920

"Experiments on the Utilization of Salep Mannan," 1920

"Some Experiments on the Digestibility of Rolled Oats Prepared in Various Ways," 1922

"The Almond as a Source of the A Vitamin," 1922

"The Basal Metabolism of Girls from Eleven to Fourteen Years of Age," 1922

"Experiments on the Utilization of the Calcium of Almonds by Man," 1923

"Digestion Experiments with the Raw White of Egg," 1923

"Maintenance Values for the Proteins of Milk, Bread-and-Milk, Meat and Soy Bean Curd in Human Nutrition," 1923

"Supplementary Values among Foods. I: Adding Egg to an Adequate Diet Compared with Increasing Vegetables," 1928

"Supplementary Values among Foods. II. Growth and Reproduction on White Bread with Various Supplements," 1928

"Studies in Nutrition. I. Growth, Reproduction, and Lactation on Diets with Different Proportions of Cereals and Vegetables," 1928

"Studies in Nutrition. II. The Effect of Adding Egg to a Diet Already Adequate," 1928

"Influence of Whole Wheat upon Hemoglobin Regeneration in Albino Rats," 1929

"The Relation of Diet to Health and Growth of Children in Institutions," 1930

"Iron Requirement in Early Childhood," 1930

"The Food Consumption of Nursery School Children," 1932

"Wheat Bran as a Source of Vitamin B," 1932

"The Influence of Bran on the Alimentary Tract," 1932

TABLE 5.1—*Continued*

"Factors in Food Influencing Hemoglobin Regeneration. I. Whole Wheat Flour, White Flour, Prepared Bran, and Oatmeal," 1932
"Factors in Food Influencing Hemoglobin Regeneration. II. Liver in Comparison with Whole Wheat and Prepared Bran," 1932
"Factors in Food Influencing Hemoglobin Regeneration. III. Eggs in Comparison with Whole Wheat, Prepared Bran, Oatmeal, Beef Liver, and Beef Muscle," 1934
"Egg Yolk and Bran as Sources of Iron in the Human Dietary," 1935
"Child Nutrition on a Low-Priced Diet: with Special Reference to the Supplementary Value of an Egg a Day, the Effect of Adding Orange Juice, and of Replacing Egg by Liver," 1935
"The Effect of Digestibility upon the Availability of Iron in Whole Wheat," 1936
"Protein Utilization as Affected by the Presence of Small Amounts of Bran or Its Fiber," 1936
"Vitamin B and G Values of Peas and Lima Beans under Various Conditions," 1937
"The Influence of Sex on Iron Utilization in Rats," 1938
"Vitamin B_1 Intake of Nursery School Children," 1938
"The Banana as a Food for the Aged," 1940

A research colleague, Professor Otis Caldwell of Teachers College and general secretary for the American Association for the Advancement of Science, spoke of her approach to scientific problems and of her procedures in research:

> In scientific work Mary Swartz Rose always made sure that she acquired accurate knowledge of the background of any particular study in which she was concerned—that is, she studied and documented the literature relating to that study. She tried to determine what is known and what is not known. She organized a clean-cut statement of the particular problems she proposed to investigate. Then she outlined a clean-cut plan of the way in which she proposed to work when making her investigation . . . she was not in any sense a chance worker, she was a guided worker: guided by her own thinking and her own studies. . . . Mrs. Rose was eminent in providing well-made plans regarding what was to be studied and how the work was to be done. As she accumulated facts she recorded them without statement or conclusions, but after she had accumulated a lot of facts she began to assemble inferences from them and to check her facts to see whether her inferences were borne out. When that was done . . . she then wanted to

> make a clean-cut statement of what changes would be made in our knowledge if the inferences were correct . . . she wanted next to make a statement of how our practice in whatever we do would be changed if her inferences were correct. When she finished a piece of work, the next student who undertook a related problem could gain from her work a summary of what was known in that field, up to the time she had attacked it, and what seemed to be known at the close of her period of work. In that sense she was a safe builder of the scientific foundations of our knowledge of nutrition as related to the welfare of children. . . .[4]

Being aware of the limitations of knowledge in the science of nutrition, Rose persuaded Teachers College authorities to equip laboratories to provide students and staff with an opportunity to carry on original research. A description of the first facilities was given in chapter 4. These were adequate for some time. Class enrollments were small in the early days. Until 1913 there was only one assistant, Mary McCormick, who had been appointed in 1911. As the number of students and staff increased through the years, interest in research in nutrition grew steadily and additional well-equipped laboratories were set up.

The establishment of the program leading to the doctor of philosophy degree in nutrition gave impetus to research in nutrition at Teachers College. This was the first Ph.D. degree that was especially planned and called nutrition in the United States. Both Grace MacLeod (1924) and Ella McCollum Vahlteich (1930) had received their doctoral degrees in chemistry rather than in nutrition although each had written nutrition dissertations. A subcommittee on nutrition, part of the Joint Committee on Graduate Instruction, composed of Sherman and two other professors in his department of chemistry along with Rose and MacLeod, was set up to be responsible for the work and dissertation for the new Ph.D. degree in nutrition. Lan-Chen Kung was the first student to receive this degree in 1932 (table 5.2).

THE ALBINO RAT AS A TOOL IN NUTRITION RESEARCH

The albino rat had been discovered to be a good deputy for humans in nutrition research by the time that Rose started her research at Teachers College. E. V. McCollum in the College of Agriculture, University of Wisconsin, had established during the academic year

TABLE 5.2 Nutrition Dissertations for the Ph.D. Degree

FACULTY OF PURE SCIENCE		
1924	MacLeod, Grace	"Studies of the Normal Basal Energy Requirement"
1930	Vahlteich, Ella McCollum	"A Quantitive Study of the Influence of Nutrients on Hemoglobin Regeneration"
JOINT COMMITTEE OF GRADUATE INSTRUCTION		
1932	Kung, Lan-Chen	"The Influence of Some Nutrients on Hemoglobin Production and the Iron Content of the Body"
1933	Potgieter, Martha	"The Energy Costs of Some Forms of Physical Activity of Nine-Year-Old Girls"
1934	Robb, Elda	"The Energy Requirement of Normal Three- and Four-Year-Old Children under Standard Basal Metabolism Conditions and during Periods of Quiet Play"
1934	Williams, Dorothy E.	"The Influence of Sleep on the Energy Metabolism of Three- and Four-Year-Old Children"
1935	Funnell, Esther, H.	"An Investigation of Vitamin B and Vitamin G Values in Some Seeds Used as Food"
1936	Hubbell, Helen Jackson	"An Investigation of the Influence of Sex on the Utilization of Iron"
1937	Taylor, Clara Mae	"The Energy Metabolism and Mechanical Efficiency of Young Boys"
1940	Thompson, Ethel M.	"A Study of the Energy Expenditure and Mechanical Efficiency of Young Girls and Adult Women"
1940	Kunerth, Bernice L.	"The Effect upon Iron Utilization of Varying Calcium and Phosphorus within the Limits of Normal Dietaries"

1907–08 the first rat colony in America for nutrition studies, undaunted by his dean's adverse decision. At first McCollum used wild rats but they were too ferocious. He then purchased a dozen albino rats from a pet stock dealer in Chicago, paying for them himself.[5, 6] In 1909 L. B. Mendel and T. B. Osborne had started their colony of albino rats at Yale University, the second of its kind in the United States.

During 1918 Mendel gave Rose two young albino rats to start a colony at Teachers College. At the end of the academic year it appeared that the newly started colony would need to be destroyed because there was no one at Teachers College to look after the animals during the summer. Sherman, however, suggested that his children care for them during the summer with the understanding that he

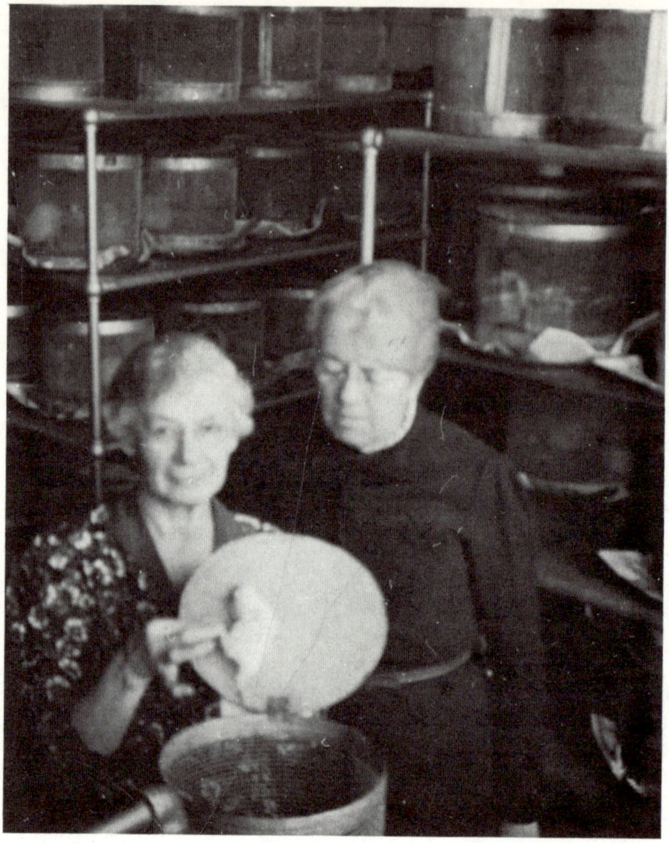

Fig. 5.1 Mary Swartz Rose and Grace MacLeod in the animal laboratory at Teachers College

have half the young rats born during the summer to start his own colony. By September there were 28 young rats for Sherman and 28 for Rose. Rose's colony was used for demonstration and teaching purposes until 1925 when it was first used for research. The colony soon outgrew the small animal laboratory on the fifth floor and was moved to larger quarters on the fourth floor (fig. 5.1). The colony was continued over fifty years until Orrea F. Pye retired.

ENERGY METABOLISM

Until 1909 the method of measuring energy was direct calorimetry involving costly, cumbersome, and time-consuming equipment. In 1908 the Nutrition Laboratory of the Carnegie Institution of Washington was established in Boston. During the next decades Director F. G. Benedict and his staff proved very ingenious in devising simpler methods and equipment to determine energy indirectly. Portable respiration apparatus and respiration chambers became available. The nutrition program at Teachers College always had a close relationship with the investigators at the Carnegie Institution at Boston. Rose had arranged for Grace MacLeod to go there to learn about energy methods and equipment. When the Carnegie Institution was finally closed a good deal of equipment was given to Taylor and Pye along with copies of the institution's voluminous publications.

Mary Swartz Rose became interested in investigating energy expenditure about 1920. Grace MacLeod had returned to Teachers College as an instructor in nutrition and was continuing her studies toward the Ph.D. degree in chemistry at Columbia. At Rose's suggestion, MacLeod began research on the basal metabolism of girls eleven to fourteen years of age. As MacLeod has said:

> I was investigating basal metabolism of young girls just because I was interested, not with the thought of using it for my dissertation towards the degree at Columbia University, where I had already matriculated for the degree of Doctor of Philosophy. When I had gathered quite a bit of data, Dr. Sherman asked if I would be willing to present my work to the chemistry faculty at Columbia University to see if they would accept it. . . . A dissertation on such a subject had never before been presented. . . . The whole committee was interested. . . . and that is how I came to do my dissertation on energy metabolism instead of in chemistry.[7]

In the early investigations, portable respiration apparatus (fig. 5.2) was used in the nutrition laboratory and in some of the rooms of the apartment on the fifth floor.

The apartment kitchen was used for the preparation of food for subjects in the research projects. The former apartment bathroom was made over and equipped for basal metabolism studies on albino rats and as a gas analysis room. The work on the basal metabolism of the rat began in 1921 and continued for about five years.

Three doctoral students (Martha Potgieter, Elda Robb, and Dorothy E. Williams) conducted metabolic research with children in the Child Development Institute of Teachers College. A respiration chamber was set up there to study: (1) energy costs of nine-year-old girls while resting, standing still, climbing stairs, and in quiet play while seated;

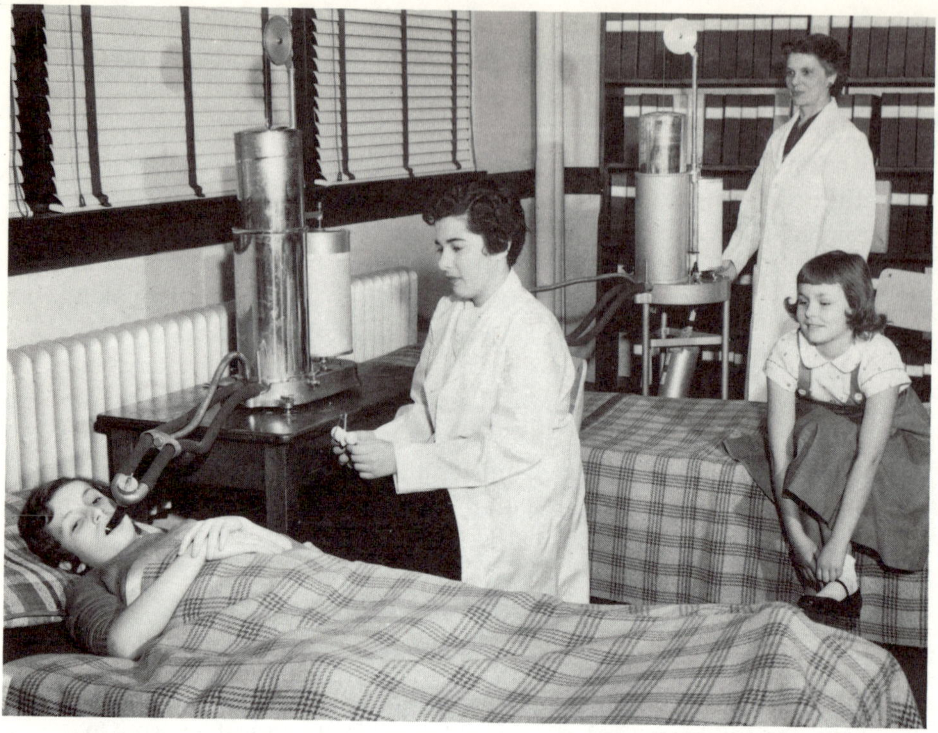

Fig. 5.2 Preparation for the measurement of basal metabolism using portable respiration apparatus

(2) energy requirement of three- and four-year-old girls and boys under basal metabolism conditions and during different types of quiet play; (3) basal metabolism and energy expenditure during an afternoon nap and immediately after waking of three- and four-year-old girls and boys.

In 1934 the respiration chamber was moved to the nutrition laboratory at Teachers College (see fig. 5.2). Clara Mae Taylor determined the basal metabolism of nine- to eleven-year-old boys by using a portable respiration apparatus and the newly installed respiration chamber that was equipped with a bicycle ergometer. She wanted to find the mechanical efficiency and energy expenditure of these boys while bicycling and for periods of quiet play while sitting. Ethel M. Thompson used the same apparatus for the study of basal metabolism, mechanical efficiency, and energy expenditure while bicycling and in seated, quiet activities of nine- to eleven-year-old girls and twenty-one- to twenty-eight-year-old women.

Energy expenditure continued to be a major aspect of research in nutrition at Teachers College during the times that MacLeod, Taylor, and Pye were in charge of the program and resulted in the accumulation and publication of much useful data.

PROTEIN AND BIOLOGICAL AVAILABILITY

In an article with Mendel in 1910 following Swartz's dissertation research, the point was made that it was common practice to look upon chemical analyses of a food material as an adequate index of its nutritive value.[8] Although these data were reliable in some cases, they were not in others because of the digestibility of a food and other factors. The authors mentioned the estimation of protein on the basis of content as likely to lead to erroneous conclusions yet that method was still in use after Rose's death.

Rose conducted studies of the biological efficiency of protein, as well as other nutrients, in numerous foods with human subjects, usually college women, and later with albino rats. Rose was interested in how digestibility and nutritive value might be affected by different methods of preparing foods. She tried out raw and cooked eggs and cereals prepared in various ways. She appreciated the supplementary values among foods such as wheat and milk. She recognized the superiority of the proteins of egg and milk over those of meat. Even in 1922 Rose had the vision to comment in an article, "In conclusion, it may be said that our newer knowledge of nutrition should make us appreciative of the fact that all dietary essentials—energy, protein, vitamins, mineral constituents—must be considered in relation to one another, none being able to function fully without the others in suitable proportions."[9] Over the years there has been a tendency to focus in research on one kind of nutrient, first energy and protein, then dramatically on vitamins, then minerals. Only recently are interrelationships among nutrients being emphasized.

STUDIES OF MINERAL ELEMENTS

The importance that Sherman attached to the mineral elements has been indicated already in the discussion of his textbook published in 1911 (see page 52). He believed that the then prevalent custom of speaking of the ash of food as if it were a more or less homogeneous substance was wholly illogical and incorrect. He stated that in comparing nutritive values, foods must not only supply fuel but also the building materials among which nitrogen, calcium, phosphorus, and iron appear to require special consideration.[10]

In 1913 Mendel and Osborne had written that animal cells needed suitable constructive materials to replace the wear and tear therein.[11] Interest in mineral elements was overshadowed by the vitamins for several years following this. In 1918, however, Osborne and Mendel, calling attention to the paucity of knowledge of minerals, wrote: "There is no adequate experimental basis whatever to permit tenable statements regarding the indispensability or even the minimum requirement of any of the inorganic constituents of the dietary with the possible exception of calcium and phosphorus."[12]

Anton Rose had received his Ph.D. degree in biological chemistry at Columbia University in 1912. He remained at Columbia in the department of chemistry for several years and carried out research in the mineral elements with Sherman, and continued his interest after he joined the staff of Prudential Insurance Company.

Is it any wonder that Mary Swartz Rose was interested in the mineral elements, particularly in iron? These three men who meant so much to her—Mendel her professor, Sherman her colleague, and Anton Rose her husband—and who all valued her abilities, stimulated her interest in the field. It is not difficult to imagine the inspiration and great satisfaction that the two Roses, scientists of equal stature and success, generated in each other.

Anton Rose and Sherman studied the phosphorus requirement of maintenance in man in 1912, and reported this and several similar unrecorded experiments in 1920.[13] From the data of ninety-two experiments it appeared that the phosphorus requirement for 70 kilograms of body weight per day ranged from 0.52 to 1.20 grams, with an average of 0.88 grams and that possibly the nature of the phosphorus compounds of intake was of more significance than usually assumed at that time.

Sherman, in cooperation with Anton Rose and Mary Swartz Rose, published in 1920 a summary of data from experiments to determine the calcium requirement of maintenance in man.[14] These ninety-seven experiments had been carried out in either Sherman's or Mary Swartz Rose's laboratory. Data indicated the calcium requirement per 70 kilograms of body weight per day ranged from 0.27 to 0.82 grams, with an average of 0.45 grams. Of interest is the closeness of the values for phosphorus and calcium to the bases of the present Recommended

Dietary Allowances. The authors stated that in the past the calcium requirement of the body had been underestimated because of the use of diets furnishing so little calcium that the output, although greater than the intake, had been depressed below the point at which equilibrium could actually be maintained.

Mendel (with H. B. McClugage) in 1918 had called attention to the scantiness of knowledge concerning the value of calcium in vegetables for animal nutrition. In the early 1920s, research was conducted at Teachers College on the utilization of the calcium of carrots and of almonds by humans. Results indicated that the calcium in carrots is well utilized and could be of value in helping to meet calcium requirements. The calcium of almonds was not found to be as well utilized as that of milk or carrots.[15, 16]

Rose's publications include reports of research on food sources of iron, iron requirements of children and adults, iron utilization, and hemoglobin regeneration by humans and by albino rats. As a student who received her Ph.D. in 1936 (Helen Jackson Hubbell) said:

> My subject—iron—was in one of Mrs. Rose's favorite fields of research. . . . Mrs. Rose worked right in the laboratory with us whenever we had a problem and needed help. In my case, as in others, when I had a new problem in technique, such as the photoelectric scopometer, she would always stand by, and so would Dr. MacLeod. Mrs. Rose always said, "Techniques in research are important. The sooner they are mastered, the more effective and interesting will be the work, the sooner the work will get under way, and from my point of view, the more reliable will be the results.[17]

Iron requirements of adult males had been established by Sherman. A number of experiments of iron balance in infants had been carried out, but none in young children over a year old until Rose and her coworkers studied them.

In Rose's laboratory, various foods, such as whole wheat flour, white flour, prepared bran, oatmeal, eggs, liver, and beef, were studied as sources of iron and as factors influencing hemoglobin regeneration. In an investigation started in 1928 it was observed that it was impossible to induce anemia in adult albino rats unless they were exclusively restricted to milk.[18] Subsequent studies showed that it was necessary to use twice as much iron in the form of liver as of whole wheat to get the same increase in hemoglobin in a six-week period in albino rats. Certain factors were noted to have influence: The form in which the iron is held in liver, and to a lesser extent in egg yolk, was a limiting factor in hemoglobin regeneration (that is, the first limiting factor in egg yolk is copper, the second limiting factor is the form in which the iron occurs, and there is a third unknown factor). Female rats stored more iron than males.[19, 20, 21] It was found that the iron of egg yolk and of bran when fed as part of a simple mixed diet can be used with equal efficiency for the maintenance of iron equilibrium in adult humans under the conditions of the experiment.[22]

Bernice Kunerth (now Watt) studied the effect of calcium and phosphorus on iron utilization, and found that both iron content and hemoglobin regeneration were depressed in albino rats when the diet contained either very high amounts of calcium and phosphorus or a moderate amount of calcium and low phosphorus.

Over fifty years ago, Rose pointed out that foods must be studied not merely in regard to total iron, but in regard to other factors in the food influencing hemoglobin formation. The accuracy of this insight has been borne out ever since by multiple studies demonstrating how many factors affect iron availability and utilization in the body. In Rose's longitudinal study of nursery school children at the Child Development Institute at Teachers College, the children were kept under constant supervision for periods up to twenty-four to thirty-two months. At the day nursery, food intake was accurately controlled. Close contact with the home made possible study of other foods eaten. Investigation indicated that the iron intake was above the estimated requirements at that time. Matched into two groups for age and other conditions as closely as possible, one group received an egg daily added to the diet, the other no egg. At the end of two years the group having the egg showed an improvement in both hemoglobin and red cell count. Another study with calves liver (total iron equal to that in egg) produced a more rapid rise in hemoglobin, but it was observed that this initial stimulus effect was lost as the study continued. Hence, Rose decided that "the egg appears to be a very valuable reinforcement for the diet of the young child."[23]

A few of the children in the above study were subjects for balance investigations of iron requirement. One three-year-old girl was studied for twelve days. The basic diet was the usual one for the child, excluding one egg daily. The average daily iron intake was 4.64 milligrams for the three nine-day balance periods with the child in negative balance averaging –1.10 milligrams. Rose estimated the subject's minimum requirement to be about 5.70 milligrams. Rose believed this was not quite adequate for the child's total needs and recommended about 0.8 milligrams iron per 100 calories to maintain equilibrium and provide for growth. It is of interest to note that the 1974 Recommended Dietary Allowances of the National Research Council suggest 15 milligrams iron and 1,300 kilocalories for the average child of one to three years, or 0.86 milligrams per 100 kilocalories.[24]

Follow-up animal studies were conducted as stated "to extend the study over a longer period of life than is possible with human beings." Rats were fed through four generations "three diets suitable for young children," differing only in the relative proportions of cereal and vegetables. Adding egg to a diet brought improvement in lactation as well as greater growth of young rats, earlier maturity of female rats, and a larger number of females bearing young. Hemoglobin and erythrocyte counts indicated that all diets fed the rats gave adequate values with or without added egg.[25]

In 1972 (more than thirty years after Rose's death), Bing pointed out that there is disagreement about the best food sources of iron and the best iron compounds for fortifying food. He recommends that educators follow the teachings of the 1930s because the older assay methods, as practiced by Rose and her collaborators, appear to be more reliable than the newer.[26]

VITAMIN RESEARCH

Mary Swartz Rose had been impressed by the first nutrition problem assigned to her as a student in the early 1900s: to provide food for a man for ten cents a day that would yield 150 grams protein, 150 grams fat, and 360 grams carbohydrate. To get sufficient protein was the objective. Calories could be taken for granted since they would be derived from the protein, fat, and carbohydrate. "Ash" was supposed to take care of itself. Vitamins were unheard of.

By 1920 three vitamins (A, B, and C) had been officially recognized and their physiological properties defined. Sherman, however, felt that it had not been proven that any one of the three stood for a single substance. There was much confusion until the vitamins were chemically separated, especially the B complex factors.

Rose and coworkers investigated certain foods as sources of vitamins and also studied the vitamin intake of young children. A doctoral student (Esther Funnell, now Phipard) studied the effects of cooking, freezing, maturing, and sprouting on the vitamin B and G content of fresh raw peas and lima beans, using growth in albino rats as a criterion, during 1933–34.[27] An analytical study of the dietaries of boys 40 to 55 months of age showed that the standard proposed as a basis of selection of food for nursery school children will furnish adequate vitamin B_1 provided at least 40 percent of the calories are derived from milk, 18 to 20 percent from cereals (at least half as whole grain products) and 16 to 22 percent from fruits and vegetables (including the daily use of 3 to 4 ounces of orange juice or equivalent tomato juice).[28]

STUDENT PROJECTS

The laboratory in Room 401 was fully equipped in the autumn of 1909. Research on foods was carried out: the weighing of foods, the calculation of dietaries, the preparation of meals. The laboratories on the fifth floor were also used from the very beginning. Students served as subjects for some investigations and small animals for others. A student in the first class (Mary McCormick) said:

> In 1909–10, I worked in the research laboratory up under the roof on the fifth floor. The problem on which I worked was the influence of nuts on the output of uric acid in the urine.[29]

Another student (Louise McD. Browne) reported:

> For my master's thesis in 1911–13 I undertook a feeding problem on the digestibility of salep mannan. . . . A graduate student . . . agreed to eat the experimental diet with me. . . . Mrs. Rose directed my work, and Dr. Sherman came over occasionally to discuss laboratory technique.[30]

A 1913 student-researcher (Lucy H. Gillett) wrote:

> I took as much work with Mrs. Rose as possible, most of which was of graduate rank. This included research to throw some light on the utilization of mannóse by the rabbit. . . . During the first years of class work with Mrs. Rose, most of us stood in awe of her quick and accurate mind and the high standard she set for our own attainments; but when we

> began the more intimate association made possible through research work, her cheerful greeting as she entered the laboratory, her real interest in our animals, and her patience with our reluctance in handling such strange educational tools made us appreciate her warmth and friendliness. . . . Mrs. Rose spent much time in our laboratory, for she seemed as interested in our rabbits as though she were watching the growth of a baby. Her unlimited vitality and method of attacking problems were always inspiring. Her questions, sometimes abrupt to be sure, would go to the root of our problems, and then a kind word and a hearty laugh would dispel the tension.[31]

In memories of early laboratory days (1915) a student (Lenna F. Cooper) recalled:

> The work that had been done by early investigators . . . suggested to us the desirability of investigating more fully the nutritive value of potato nitrogen . . . under carefully controlled conditions and determining how quickly nitrogen equilibrium could be established. . . . I feel that I got more out of my research because I had the personal guidance of Mrs. Rose throughout the experiment. . . . The foundations for much of my work later on were laid in that laboratory.[32]

DIETARY STUDIES

Mary Swartz Rose was very interested in the nutrition of children—in finding out what foods they were eating, how their diets could be evaluated, what standards should be established for feeding children, what should be taught to children about foods, and what mothers and other people responsible for the child's food should know about nutrition.

Her concern with the evaluation of diets led her in 1911 to study four- to twenty-one-year-old children hospitalized for diseases of the bone but leading fairly normal lives. Diets were analyzed for cost, energy value, protein, phosphoric acid, lime, and iron. A score was given for each individual item and a value derived. Findings indicated that when the food score was numerically higher than the percentage of cost of the food, that food could be regarded as a comparatively inexpensive item in the diet and a better buy than if the reverse were true. For example, milk had a food score of 27 and cost 19 percent of all foods while meats and fish with a food score of only 18 cost 25 percent of the total cost of food. An allowance was made for kitchen and table waste, 20 percent for the hospital because less use can be made of table waste in an institution than in a family home where a loss of 10 percent was considered as not unusual.[33] This method of dietary analysis received favorable comments from Lafayette B. Mendel (see fig. 3.4.)

Research was started in the late 1920s to discover whether the study of a dietary by food groups and the determination of percent of kilocalories furnished by each group would be valuable in finding defects in the quality of the dietary. Dietaries in four child-caring institutions were studied, all but one being continued for a year. The six food groups selected were: (1) foods from cereal grains, (2) milk, (3) fruits and vegetables, (4) fats and oils, (5) sugars and sweets, (6) eggs, cheese, meats, and other flesh foods. It was found that the percentages of kilocalories provided by the food groups did reveal probable defects in the diet.[34]

A quantitative dietary study was made of children in a nursery school, using the six food groups, to determine what children under two and a half years of age and children two and a half to four years of age were eating. Cost of food was not a factor in this situation, and the intake of fruits and vegetables was found to be higher, and cereals lower, than in other reported studies. Fat intake, true today also, was found to be too high for some children in these well-to-do families. In some cases sugar was unsuitably high due to its too generous use with cereal. Also true over forty-five years later! Those children with a distribution of calories approximating the median values found for each food group had an excellent dietary, adequate in protein, calcium, phosphorus, and vitamins (insofar as was known then about vitamins), but maybe not as high in iron and vitamin B as further investigation might prove desirable. As an outcome of this study, a new standard for distribution of foods to nursery school children was suggested:[35]

Cereal grains	18–20% of total calories
Milk	45–55
Fruits and vegetables	16–22
Fats	4–8
Sugar	1–3
Eggs and meat	3–5

Rose continued her research with children throughout her lifetime. She believed that good nutrition in the child begins with the mother. Research with experimental animals had proven that withholding certain elements from an adequate diet interfered with normal reproduction in the animal. Although the greatest single dietary cause of malnutrition in children was an inadequate supply of total food, Rose felt that protein, ash constituents, and vitamins were also required for growth. She cooperated in research in the Child Development Institute, with various departments of the college, and with a social welfare agency for many years. She conducted research in the institute in metabolism, nutrition education, and adequacy of diets, especially in relation to iron.

Rose's final scientific research, which she published, was carried out in six homes for the elderly. She believed that diets for the elderly should be more like those for the young in their content of protective foods than had been formerly thought necessary. Findings of her study revealed that bananas were well liked and digested without difficulty by people beyond sixty-five years of age. And, aside from citrus fruits and tomatoes, there are few foods easily eaten by old people which will furnish as much vitamin C as a banana.[36] Today older people, especially those on diuretics, are advised to take bananas for another nutrient—potassium.

We cannot begin our nutrition teaching too early—MSR

chapter six ROSE'S CONTRIBUTIONS TO NUTRITION EDUCATION IN THE SCHOOL

SOME HISTORICAL ASPECTS OF NUTRITION EDUCATION

Mary Swartz Rose always emphasized the importance of good nutrition during the growing years. She recognized that it is more difficult to change behavior after habits are formed than before they become established. She, therefore, placed special emphasis on the need for nutrition teaching in the early school years and the necessity for continuing this teaching throughout the school years by providing education appropriate to the age and understanding of the child. For many years she applied her creative imagination and her meticulous research methods to the study of nutrition education in the school, particularly in the elementary school.

Speaking on nutrition and health of the school child, Rose made a number of points:

- I believe in the optimum diet for every child.
- I believe in the education of the community to the school lunch as an integral part of the educational program.

• I believe in the education of teachers to cooperate in the school nutrition program and to uphold the cafeteria manager in her efforts to provide a lunch of high protective value.[1]

She did not, of course, foresee the political use and commercialization of the school lunch as in our day. She anticipated a well-trained nutrition person working in the school lunch whose primary concern was the nutrition of the school child and also well-informed teachers who could reinforce in the classroom the good nutrition principles demonstrated in the school lunch.[2]

Historically, nutrition education in the school goes back a long time. G. J. Mulder (1802–80), whose name is linked with proteins because he introduced the term in 1838, was interested in several aspects of human nutrition. He advocated the teaching of nutrition in the regular schools, but his proposal was not accepted. He was ahead of his time.[3]

In this country, Ellen H. Richards, emphasized the importance of the school lunch[4] and expressed the belief that the school noon hour should be utilized for social training and the acquirement of good habits.[5]

Shortly after Mary Swartz Rose's return to Teachers College in 1909 she began to write in various publications articles on child nutrition directed to different groups in the population: parents and families, lay and professional groups, teachers of various kinds, and nutritionists and dietitians. Her first publication about food for young children was in 1911.[6] Rose pointed out that if children are to have useful bodies and minds they must be given the right kind of food at the proper time.

She advocated regularity of mealtimes for children and the avoidance of giving food too often and meals too close together. Milk was considered the best food for children of all ages, and emphasis was placed on bread, whole grain cereals (fig. 6.1), eggs, fruit (even bananas, which many people in 1911 considered harmful for children), fresh vegetables, and a liberal amount of water. Meat was not recommended for children under eight years of age if eggs and milk were provided. It was felt that eggs and milk were better sources of protein (and other nutrients) for children than meat.

Mrs. Rose didn't think that children needed to be introduced to meat. Mrs. Rose felt that there were two reasons for introducing foods to children: (1) for nutrition and (2) for introducing foods whose taste

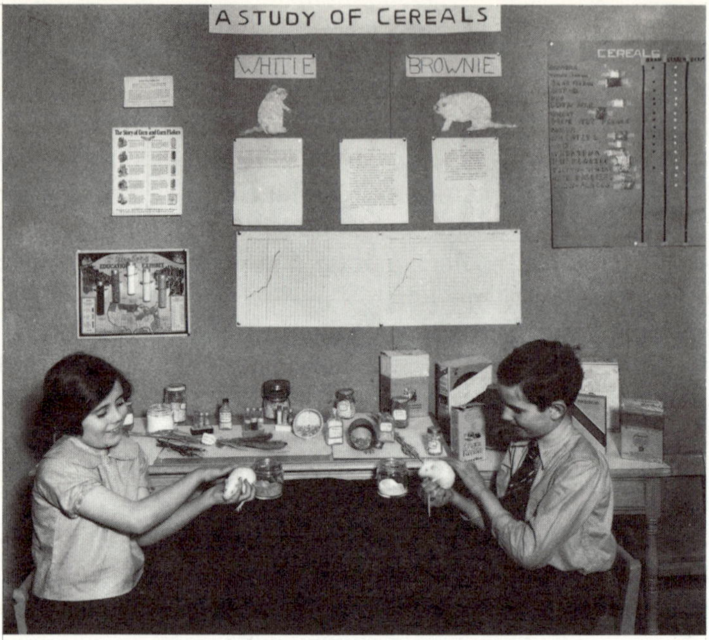

Fig. 6.1 A study of cereals

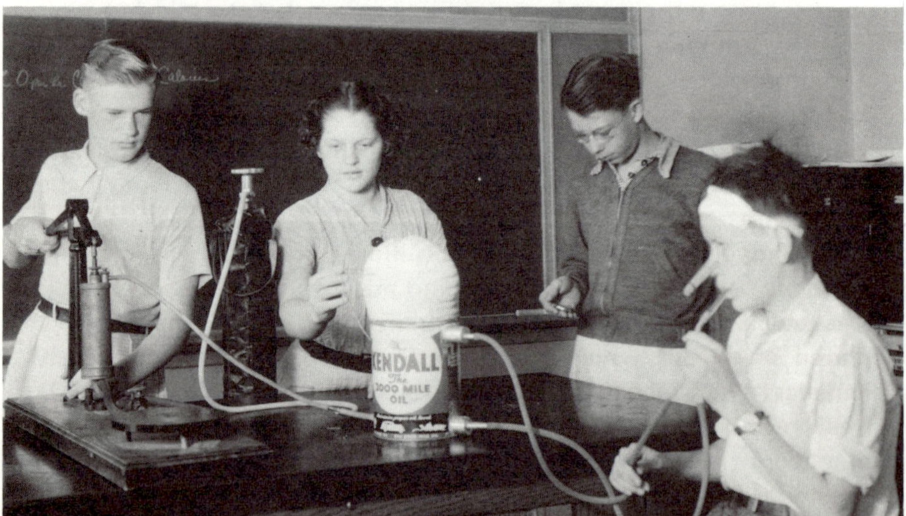

Fig. 6.2 Homemade respiration apparatus constructed and used by high school students in their biology courses. Nutrition work in the biology classes was under Rose's guidance.

they might not like. Since she believed that everybody liked the taste of meat, she saw no reason for introducing it to the young child. For older children, meat cooked without fat and fish free from fat were suggested. Menus for children of different ages and for children who would not drink milk were given with the nutritive value and cost.

Rose's first publication on lessons in food and nutrition was in 1917.[7] The scope of her interest in this area is indicated by the titles of her publications (table 6.1). Rose conducted research in public and private schools in New York City and in schools outside the city, particularly in Edgewater and Glen Rock, New Jersey. She cooperated in the development of courses for schools in areas such as Newark, New Jersey, and Westfield, Massachusetts (fig. 6.2). She worked with teachers from several school districts in Long Island, New York. Clara Mae Taylor was associated with Rose in many of the school programs over the years.

In reporting on her first nutrition classes held in conjunction with a public school (P. S. 43, New York City), Rose wrote:

> A glass of sugar syrup stands fluid and transparent. Into it a few sugar crystals are dropped. With this seeding the whole glass becomes soon a solid mass of crystals. How could so slight an addition have so profound an effect? The social world seems often like a glass of sugar syrup. Forces accumulate, and some special movement, small in itself, gives a totally new aspect to the situation. . . . What has happened thus at large seems typical of what has taken place at P.S. 43. It had the usual health equipment of a public school—medical inspector, visiting nurse, home economics teachers for the 7th and 8th grades—and what is less usual, a visiting teacher to make close connection with the homes. Much was done, but everybody knew much remained to be done to eliminate the present and potential handicap of undernutrition and to fortify the child with first class health habits.
>
> Into this solution fell a few crystals also. I think I may justly say that one of the first was the Morningside Nutrition Center. When that subcommittee of three from the larger Home Economics Committee of the Charity Organization Society gathered together at the Henry Street Branch on Amsterdam Avenue—a group of social workers representing the neighborhood—no one visualized the work now inaugurated in the school. Some of us were bent on providing a training school in which home economics students might learn to make their technical knowledge available to the community, and some of us were bent on securing help for the child or family here and there whom no other

organization was quite equipped to deal with. But we drew our first nutrition class from P. S. 43. We met in that old saloon, and sang a health to milk.

> Here's to your good health and mine,
> To make us grow this milk is fine:
> A cup a morn, at evening, too,
> To bring good health to me and you.

Mrs. Mudge brought her ukulele, and because of the hum inside had to retreat to the street to tune it! . . . We were very happy at the little Morningside Center. We were busy studying the educational and social problems involved in children's nutrition classes for different ages, in classes for the mothers of the neighborhood and in the training of students. In the year and a half we were there we came into contact with over 175 families and gave 89 students training which has resulted in most of them continuing the work elsewhere in some form or other.

But great as the possibilities were, our resources were very limited. So we appealed to . . . the outcome of which was crystallization of a coordinated health program for the school. . . . With this assistance the Morningside Center was equipped to organize nutrition classes in the school. . . . This cooperative health enterprise was started in the school the first of February. . . .

On the educational side, we think that we have found out from our previous experience some of the things which it is profitable to try to do. Lessons are necessarily short but each has a definite topic. . . . Food lessons are first centered around specific food which should be a regular part of the child's diet—those which he should know, respect and like. At the Morningside Center we were fully convinced that the serving of food has a distinct value in these children's classes. It not only interested the children at the time, but it made a much deeper impression than merely talking about it, so that they were more likely to tell about it at home. . . . Besides teaching the common foods children should eat and like, we try to teach something about meals. . . .

While we lost something of the freedom of the "Lawrence Club," as the children called it, by moving into the school, we have this advantage of closer contact with the teachers, as well as the opportunity to hold more classes than we could have in our small center after school hours.[8]

While the work just described was being carried out with children of a public school, Rose was also studying nutrition education of children in a different type of setting. During the summer of 1919, she conducted a nutrition class in the clinic organized for the seventy-five malnourished children attending the summer play school at Stuyvesant Neighborhood House on the lower East Side of New York City. Many mothers as well as the children attended the weekly classes. Twenty-five nutrition students from Rose's classes at Teachers College were each assigned three children, visiting their homes weekly, attending them while going to the clinic, and preparing weight charts. Rose pointed out that this type of work was in its infancy.[9] She referred to the work by Lydia J. Roberts with the "individual method" and the "class method" of nutrition education in a clinic situation at the Central Free Dispensary of Rush Medical College, Chicago, in 1918. Rose also mentioned her indebtedness to W. R. Emerson and Charles H. Smith for demonstrating the power of group rivalry as an incentive to proper eating and other habits essential to normal growth in children. In 1908 Emerson had developed in Boston the first nutrition class in a clinic situation in the United States. Smith, following Emerson's methods, had set up nutrition classes with undernourished children in New York at Bellevue Hospital and at P.S. 40.[10]

ROSE'S WORK IN THE SCHOOL

At Teachers College, Rose was in an academic setting where experts were available to offer advice and cooperation whenever needed. She served on educational research institutes at the college where her colleagues found her a dynamic and stimulating participant. Her early teaching experience in schools stood her in good stead in offering practical suggestions in teaching children.

Rose, with the research worker's approach, began her studies of how to teach nutrition to school girls and boys with classes of twelve to eighteen children. Each class was taught by a student of nutrition at Teachers College, under Rose's supervision insofar as the lessons were concerned and under the immediate direction of the two nutrition workers at the school, one of whom supervised the home visiting done in connection with the classes. Rose believed that the nutrition class gave to children in groups instruction which might be meted out to them privately and individually in a nutrition clinic, and, it had the advantage of being able to help children who are not apt to go to a hospital clinic.[11] In successive years she experimented with materials and methods, the lessons being continuously extended and enriched until they were published in 1932 as *Teaching Nutrition to Boys and Girls,* the first nutrition book directed at effective teaching methods and materials for the elementary school. In the preface of this book, Rose stated:

> Instead of being a matter of accident, impulse, or whim, eating should be guided by intelligence as to the nutritive properties of foods. But if nutrition is thus to guide eating habits it must begin to function as soon as habits begin to form. At first, then, control is in the hands of the adults who care for the baby and it is their obligation to see that he learns to eat foods which promote health and growth at regular times, and with good emotional attitudes. As the child grows, his own choice must be directed so that he will eventually be able to deal wisely with his appetite and make habitually profitable selections of food for himself. Ten years of study of the teaching of nutrition in all grades from kindergarten to the eighth has made it quite evident that the first level at which some clearly formulated nutrition principles may be most profitably developed with children is about the fourth or fifth grade. This is the time when children begin to be interested in control of their own lives, and also when they are often given increasing latitude in choice of their food.
>
> But nutrition is not a simple science. It can be successfully taught only by the same careful selection and adaptation of subject matter which characterize other school subjects, such as arithmetic or history. The lessons for the intermediate grades which are described in this little book have been evolved in the process of teaching many groups of children in an elementary school.[12]

The early food lessons for children from eight to ten years old were reported in 1922, not with the idea that they were the only kind practical for nutrition classes, but to give an indication of the most suitable subject matter and the best ways of presenting it. These eighteen food lessons were arranged in groups of six lessons each to make a progressive series.[13]

In 1925 publications, Rose illustrated the use of a story of the "Getsick" and "Keepwell" families as a vehicle for a term's teaching to third-grade children in a twenty-minute weekly period,[14] and the value of considering each food as a member of a "family" when teaching ten lessons to fourth grade children.[15]

In 1925 Rose and her Teachers College students began an intensive study of the teaching of food in relation to health with fifth- and

TABLE 6.1 Titles of Publications on Nutrition Education in the School, with Date of Publication

"The Training of the School Dietitian," 1912
"Food for School Boys and Girls," 1914
"Lessons on Food and Nutrition," 1917
"A Nutrition Class in Co-operation with a Summer Play School," 1920
"Recent Developments in Child Feeding," 1920
"The Child's Day: An Entertainment to Impress Daily Habits for Healthy Life," 1921
"Food Lessons for Nutrition Classes," 1922
"Teaching Nutrition to Third-Grade Children," 1924
"Nutrition in an Elementary School," 1925
"Has Nutrition Found Its Rightful Place in Education?" 1926
"The Nutrition Classes of the Health Experiment," 1926
"A Health Experiment in Miss Goodhart's Room," 1927
"Nutrition in Health Education," 1929
"A Five-Year Study of Nutrition Teaching in the Fifth and Sixth Grades of the Elementary School," 1930
"Old and New Emphases in the Teaching of Nutrition," 1930
"Our Children and Their Nutrition Needs," 1932
"Teaching Nutrition to Boys and Girls," 1932
"Good Teaching Important If Children Are to Benefit from Knowledge of Nutrition," 1938
"Our Cereals. A Nutrition Unit for the Fourth, Fifth, and Sixth Grades of the Elementary School," 1938
"Nutrition and the Health of the School Child," 1939
"A Nutrition Program for the Elementary Grades," 1939
"Diet," 1939
"Feeding Our Teeth. A Nutrition Unit for the Third and Fourth Grades of the Elementary School," 1940
"Vegetables to Help Us Grow. A Nutrition Unit for the First, Second, and Third Grades of the Elementary School," 1941

sixth-grade children. Throughout the five-year study, she stated that an attempt was made to select certain basic ideas that anyone whose life is to be guided by the science of nutrition must appreciate; to arrange these in sequence according to suitability; and by repeated tests to determine whether children can grasp them and make them a driving force in their lives. A series of ten lessons for each term centered around a single dietary essential, with its significance for health and growth stated in simple terms.[16]

Research techniques were tested as carefully in the classroom as in the laboratory. Every detail had to be considered by the Teachers College student responsible for a lesson; Rose checked the plans and, whenever possible, sat at the back of the classroom to evaluate the lesson. Written reports of each lesson included statements of subject, aim, procedures, points made, illustrative material, and assignment (if given). A review of these reports made over many years reveals the achievement of success. Although plans made were discussed thoroughly prior to the lesson, there was flexibility in carrying them out. For example, Rose in "Comments" of a particular lesson stated:

> The lesson demonstrated excellent teaching because the questions which the children brought up in class (due to their interest in the previous lesson) and their own personal problems were discussed rather than the lesson planned.[17]

And in another situation with a different student-teacher, Rose commented on the need for careful phraseology. She wrote:

> The children were quite interested in the lesson, and the showing of the rats to them outside the cage was very effective. Some questions in the lesson were not stated in such a way that the children were required to think out answers.[18]

The well-made plans, however, did not always work out as expected. On one occasion Rose commented:

> When Miss——asked about the requirement for gas in her two cars, Felix noticed that the small one was a Packard and he immediately said that it would take more gas than the larger car. Miss ——quickly substituted a picture of a Ford coupe for the picture of the small Packard.[19]

Soon after the opening of the experimental school P.S. 500, the Speyer School, conducted by the Board of Education of New York City and Teachers College, Rose started nutrition lessons in two of the classes. She was assisted by Dr. Elda Robb. These classes were so successful that in 1936 a five-year study was initiated and nutrition lessons were held once a week in all classrooms. Two types of children were accepted by this school: slow learners and gifted children. In order that the materials planned for a grade level in this school should not be limited to exceptional children, the study was extended to several other schools where the grades were made up of the usual assortment of children. Bertlyn Bosley was employed as research assistant with responsibility for the development of the entire project. She was assisted by Eloise Cofer, Emma Gardner, Katherine Nugent, and Ruth Pike. Rose required that the assistants in the project be able "to say things three ways" so that children of different abilities could understand what was being taught. Thus, Rose working with Bosley was able to formulate and test a progressive nutrition education program through the grades. In the study, teaching techniques as well as frequency of lessons were tested and homes were visited to determine the carryover of ideas. Rose stimulated a great deal of activity by these studies, not only at Teachers College but also in other places. Both Taylor and Bosley continued their interest in school programs (fig. 6.3). Bosley in the Epilogue (see page 135) writes of nutrition education in the schools.

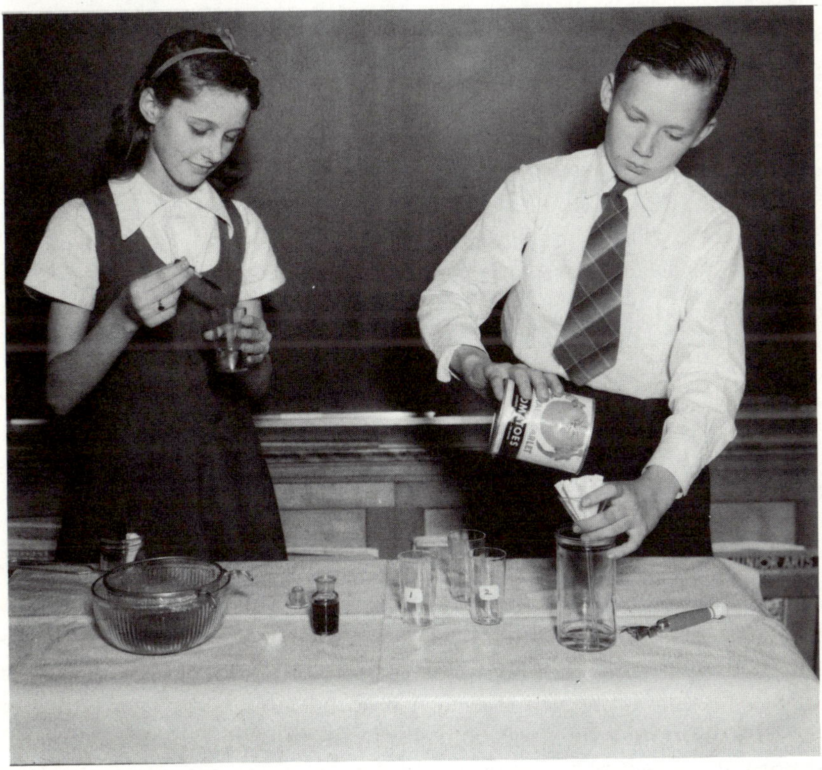

Fig. 6.3 Testing for vitamin C

Unfortunately, Rose died before the experimental work in Speyer School was completed and reported. Dr. Bosley completed it with the assistance of Professor Grace MacLeod. Three booklets were published from the five-year study.[20, 21, 22]

Rose's experimental studies in actual school settings resulted in the discovery of many innovative and valuable ways of teaching nutrition and food habit formation to children. As Todhunter has said:

> Mrs. Rose's plans and procedures are worthy of close study because current recommendations today differ little if any from these and in many places we have not yet begun to put in practice what Rose so carefully formulated from her research into methods of teaching nutrition. . . .
>
> Mrs. Rose and her group carefully selected material that was clear and vivid; the phraseology used was nutritionally accurate and at the same time full of meaning for children. She worked to find out what was the length of time needed to make each new nutritional concept clear. Mrs. Rose was practical, her keen mind saw the issues and how to reach them. She knew nutrition, but she also knew children and how to teach. . . . Her nutrition education program was based on the fact that food makes a difference in health; therefore, she taught that we need to know the kind and amount of food. Activities were the key to her nutrition education program with the children doing the talking, eating and using the foods, seeing and doing animal experiments, finding comparable illustrations in their own world and drawing their own conclusions—in other words, individual involvement.[23]

ROSE'S BELIEFS AND PRINCIPLES ON NUTRITION EDUCATION

• For further progress in nutrition and health, it is . . . essential that every potential parent, that is, every boy and girl in our schools today, learns how fundamental good nutrition is to successful living.[24]

• Nutrition has not found its rightful place in education until every child before leaving the elementary school has learned what the essentials of good nutrition are, has been helped to acquire safeguarding food habits, and has gained respect for what food can do for health.[25]

• Nutrition knowledge is complex, and must be carefully selected, graded and illuminated. Facts to be taught must relate to individual and community needs and lead to a definite and feasible course of action. "Eat wholesome food" is a futile rule, because it is too indefinite. "Eat four oranges a day" is certainly an unwise prescription when the family budget is limited and oranges are expensive. Even if the pocketbook permits and the community markets make the desirable food accessible, there may still be much inertia to overcome. The "natural" way is to eat what one pleases regardless of consequences. How shall the value of a controlled appetite be so impressed as to result in action, not once or twice, but habitually? Every bit of subject matter must not only be thoughtfully selected, but must be so presented that attitudes and ideals are developed which shall be strong enough to establish habits.[26]

• With the average child below the fourth grade, the chief aim of nutrition teaching should be to develop favorable attitudes towards foods that are needed for growing children.[27]

• The students of dietetics need to learn how to work in the public schools for this is one of the important strategic points for the instruction and nutritional care of older children.[28]

• The nutritionist must be a teacher—a very up-to-date teacher. She must be trained in education as well as in nutrition and social service. The present generation of school teachers, many of them eager to help, are impotent because they have no nutrition knowledge. The nutritionist cannot help them unless she speaks their language.[29]

Nutrition is a science of immediate application to life—MSR

chapter seven ROSE'S CONTRIBUTIONS IN EDUCATION OF THE PUBLIC

Mary Swartz Rose, it has been said, should always be remembered as one of the great interpreters of nutrition for she took the laboratory discoveries of the science and converted them to usable forms that could function in the lives of people.[1]

A philanthropic motivation seemed to have directed Mary Swartz Rose's life. This is understandable when one remembers that in the home in which she grew up the religious and charitable acts of her mother were blended with the social and reform interests of her father, and that part of her education was in institutions that fostered these ideals. She had her first contacts with domestic science at the Chautauqua Institute, a summer educational institution she attended in 1901, which offered courses in the arts, sciences, and humanities. Mechanics Institute, which she entered in the autumn of 1901, was interested in the betterment of the working person and aimed to supplement the traditional, formal education of existing colleges by its course work. There she registered for courses in domestic science because she had decided by that time to follow her interests in this new field as her life work. In addition to these influences, she lived during periods of national crisis—World War I and the great depression—which fostered a sense of responsibility.

Mary Swartz Rose had concern for the ordinary man and woman and their families and for their betterment in terms of daily living. She realized the importance of educating the homemaker in foods and nutrition and the necessity of demonstrating to people the relationship of food to health. During her lifetime, she contributed to the education of the public in nutrition through her work with organizations, through her published articles and books, and through her many contacts with people.

PARTICIPATION IN LOCAL ORGANIZATIONS

Many of the committees on which Rose served were important for their work in presenting nutrition facts to the public and in developing community nutrition programs. The first of her extracurricular activities while at Teachers College was serving as a member of the New York Milk Committee in 1909. During the following year, she had charge of planning and setting up a nutrition booth at an exhibit given by that committee.

No better example of the way in which Rose faced challenges can be found than her participation in the United States Food Administration, authorized by Congress in August 1917. Herbert Hoover was named head of the organization and Mary Swartz Rose deputy director of the Bureau of Food Conservation of the Federal Food Board and the New York State Food Commission. The functions of the bureau included the promotion of public education in the uses, preparation, substitution, and saving of foods. The bureau applied the national program in appropriate ways to the local situation by arranging publicity; furnishing speakers; preparing and publishing literature; conducting demonstrations in individual homes and in public buildings and at group meetings; setting up exhibits, sometimes accompanied by talks; and investigating methods of conserving foods where there was a scarcity and using foods when there was a surplus.

Her organizational ability, her perseverance tempered with a sense of humor that accepted what could not be changed, and her ability to work successfully with people are evident in comments from letters to her husband (fig. 7.1) regarding the Food Commission. She wrote on November 21, 1918:

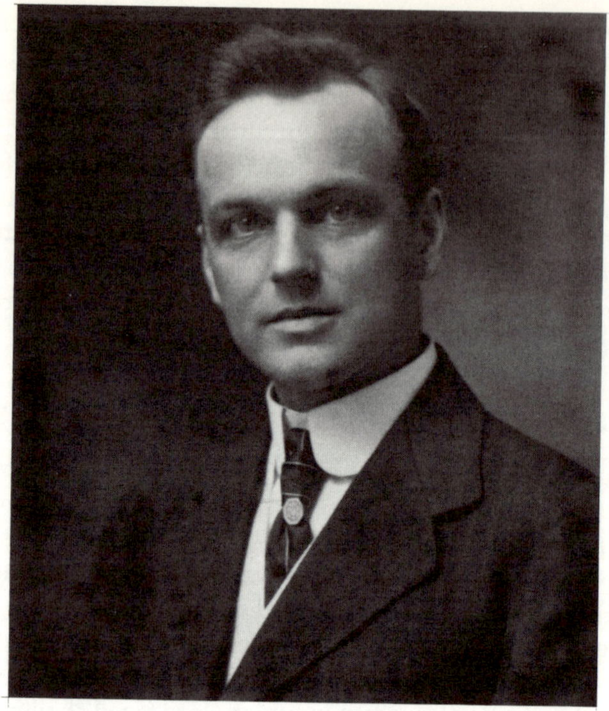

Fig. 7.1 Anton R. Rose

I went to Washington Tuesday, spent a strenuous day seeing things at the Food Administration. Among other things, I called on Mr. Ricard, who is taking Mr. Hoover's place in his absence, and presented to him the dire needs in New York City for a Conservation Exhibit, with the effect that I am now launched on another agony like that at the time of the Food Show, only I hope to profit somewhat by the former experience.

Our aim this time is to set up business on the steps of the Public Library (on Fifth Avenue). This has become quite a community center in the last three months. There is a tank and a few other little obstacles, and just how we will blow them up or overcome them I do not know. I am trying to get people together today, and our idea is to get up children in a sort of pageant effect in connection with a ship for world relief. I may be dead to the world for a few days, as we are also trying to round up all the women's clubs of the city for special programs for Conservation Week. Needless to say our office is humping.

I got back Wednesday morning and am pushing as fast as possible, because December 1st is the beginning of Conservation Week.

And on December 5th she wrote:

> Accordingly I came back and went to work. Miss Glover fortunately was here to be my mainstay. Enough said. She found a nice Mr. H, who secured for us a caravel which appeared in the Fourth of July parade, and is said to have cost one thousand dollars to build—probably true. Mr. H got it, put it in shape, put it up, and attended to innumerable details for the magnificent sum of $450. The ship secured, we went to work on space. We had learned by inquiry that it would be possible to get some space on the Library steps, but we wanted the middle space, where stands a big tank. The Tank Recruiting Corps had been given this space for the duration of the war so we set ourselves to the task of melting the heart of an officer of the Tank Corps. But the heart of the gentleman with the German name was hard and his ways were crooked. He sent us to all sorts of people who, he said, had the final word, and none of them did. Finally we got Washington on the job, and even working through the authorities at Washington, we were unable to dislocate the tank. Saturday afternoon we realized that we had met our Waterloo as far as that space was concerned, so we went to the library and consulted the Director, Mr. G, who advised us to take the space between the tank and one of the big lions. So Monday morning we went at it, finishing the details of the pageant, and at 11:30 sat back with the satisfied consciousness that everything was done. Ten minutes later I learned that there was a power above Mr. G, who would not let our ship go on the steps of the library in the space we had planned, and we had to put the ship down in front of the lion, close to the sidewalk. . . . We felt for a time weak and small. Then we gathered ourselves up, made the pageant over to fit the ship on the sidewalk, and got ready to go ahead. . . .
>
> We hold our show (lasting about fifteen minutes in actual acting) nominally at three o'clock, but it takes pretty nearly an hour to get under way. . . .
>
> The pageant is really effective. I go down every afternoon to see the beginning. There is a big crowd all over the upper library steps and the street, very quiet and attentive. . . .
>
> In all the mad rush to get this thing together, we were straining ourselves to the utmost to get out six thousand letters to the women's clubs of the city, asking them to observe yesterday as special Food Conservation Day, and in consequence of this advertising, we were called on to supply demonstrations and exhibits beyond our usual number. We have altogether at least 100 demonstrations and club meetings, and our demonstrators are taking care of about fifteen exhibits in

> libraries, church fairs, and other places. I think that this week marks the high water mark of our career.[2]

The Food Show mentioned in her letter was held in January 1918. Other food shows were held during that year, an especially large one in May. One of the food demonstrators who had worked with Rose in the Bureau of Food Conservation stated:

> I've often thought of what good psychology Mrs. Rose used in the exhibits and in all the work of the bureau.

Another said:

> We had a huge food show at Grand Central Palace, and we were all brought in to demonstrate. . . . We worked from eleven o'clock in the morning until eleven at night. Those were hard-working and busy days, and Mrs. Rose was as busy or busier than the rest of us.

A third commented:

> I remember riding home late at night from the food conservation shows. . . . After a long day spent in her office and at the college, Dr. Rose would come down to observe how effective the visual demonstration of food conservation was proving and to suggest changes when the reaction of the public indicated a lack of understanding of her purpose. If the night was very hot, the ride home would be on top of the bus, an ice cream cone apiece in hand to help lower the temperature. Only those need "Stand on their dignity" whose dignity is not innate. Hers was a patrician dignity.

And still another said:

> Mrs. Rose, a very personification of knowledge, energy, and charm, had at a week's notice prepared four booths bringing home immediately to anyone who saw them the story of the reason why we were being asked to save wheat, meat, fats, and sugar. . . . It is my belief that during the entire period of the war Mrs. Rose gave ten hours a day of concentrated service to the cause of food saving and the elimination of waste.[3]

In 1917 Mary Swartz Rose cooperated with the Life Extension Institute of New York City in demonstrating to the public that a nutritious diet costing no more than 25¢ a day could be palatable and acceptable. Rose and her assistants planned and supervised the preparation of the meals. Twenty-five young men from the City Police Department volunteered to eat the meals for a three-week period. Physical examinations showed that they had benefited from the experiment. The volunteers gave every indication of having enjoyed the meals. A final report, including menus and recipes, was published.[4,5]

In October 1920, the New York (City) Nutrition Council was founded. It was the first organization of professional people interested in nutrition as related to social and public health work. Mary Swartz Rose was named its first chairman. Committees of the council carried on many important activities. Rose assisted its Nutrition Bibliography Committee in the preparation of a nutrition bibliography published in 1921 and served as a member of the committee when it prepared the second edition of the bibliography in 1923.[6] The nutrition bibliography was prepared for the physician, organizer and supervisor of nutrition work, and field worker, nurse, teacher, and nutrition student. Rose approved all diets recommended in *Good Nutrition and Adequate Food Allowances for the Family,* a publication for executives and field workers of public health and relief organizations prepared by the Committee on Economic Standards.[7]

In 1922 Rose assisted the New York City Department of Health in formulating policies relating to food and nutrition. In 1933 she again cooperated with the department in preparing a series of six articles, with menus, enabling people to live on 50¢ a day. This series was published in daily newspapers. The information was designed to be helpful to single people who needed to economize but had no facilities for preparing food where they lived. Practically all existing information of this type was written for the housewife.[8]

Mary Swartz Rose also served as a member of several other organizations, including the advisory committee of the Association for Improving the Condition of the Poor, the governing board and chairman of the nutrition committee of the East Harlem Nursing and Health Center, the advisory committee on foods and nutrition of the Child Health Council, the advisory council to the editors of the New York Herald Tribune, and the New York Committee for Better Homes in America.

WRITINGS FOR THE PUBLIC

Rose was a prolific writer who could present the findings of her research, her evaluation or review of a topic or her beliefs and convictions in an area in either scientific or nontechnical language as the occasion demanded. In her educational publications (table 7.1), she wrote popular, semiscientific, and scientific articles and books. The popular articles were intended for the general public and were written in a direct, simple, personal style with references to everyday occurrences and to well-known stories such as *Alice in Wonderland* and *Peter Pan.* The semiscientific and scientific publications dealt with major problems, sometimes complex, in a concise, practical manner and were written frequently for the professional person interested in the health and welfare of the family.

She wrote her first popular article "How Much Meat?"[9] in 1910, that busy year during which her first scientific article was also published, and she married and established with her husband their first home in an apartment near the university.

In an early writing, "Some Facts to Help the Housewife in Feeding the Family," she described how food meets body needs, and cautioned that "some foods contain only one kind of food material and so serve only one, or possibly two, body needs. They are not bad foods on that account, but must be combined with other foods providing what they lack."[10] Still good advice today.

During the war period, she wrote several booklets and articles such as one in which suggestions were made for keeping children well and strong, with models for meals given,[11] and one in which conservation and sharing were emphasized.[12] She was author of a small book entitled *Everyday Foods in War Time.*[13] In the preface of this book she portrayed the dilemma of the housewife in trying to meet her war food needs, and she suggested "that a simple explanation of the part which some of our common foods play in our diet might be both helpful and reassuring." Included in the book were three previously published articles which she had written for *The Farmer's Wife,* October and November 1917 and June 1918: "The Milk Pitcher in the Home," "Cereals We Ought to Eat," and "Are Fruits and Vegetables Luxuries?"

In the early 1920s Rose pointed out a concept that is just as important today as it was then, namely "All dietary essentials . . . must be considered in relation to one another, none being able to function fully without the others in suitable proportions."[14]

In discussing family food habits in the 1930s, she recommended "the liberal use of milk, tomatoes, cod liver oil, green vegetables and whole grain cereals to ameliorate the evils of poverty."[15]

TABLE 7.1 Titles of Educational Publications, with Date of Publication

*"How Much Meat?" 1910
"Physiological Utilization of Some Complex Carbohydrates," 1910
†The Feeding of Young Children, 1911
"Some Problems in Dietetics", 1911
"Nutritive Value of Seaweeds," 1912
"What Anaesthesia Has Done for Surgery," 1912
Bibliographies of Home Economics Literature, nos. 1, 2, and 3, 1912
Bibliographies of Current Home Economics Literature, nos. 4 and 5, 1912
*"How a Knowledge of Food Values Will Help the Housewife to Reduce the Cost of Living," 1912
†*Feeding the Family,* 1916
†"Some Food Facts to Help the Housewife in Feeding the Family," 1916
†"Economical Diet and Cookery in Time of Emergency," 1917
†"How to Plan Meals in War Time, With Economical Menus and Suggestions for Marketing," 1917
†The Children's Food, 1917
"Redundant Sigmoid," 1917
*"Wheat Substitutes," 1917
*"The Same Nourishment for Less Money," 1917
†*Everyday Foods in War Time,* 1918
*"My Husband Won't Eat It," 1918
*"Living on Twenty-five Cents a Day," 1918
*"Team Work in Food Conservation," 1918
"On the Utilization of Salep Mannan," 1919
"The Utilization of the Calcium of Carrots by Man," 1919
"The Question of Child Feeding," 1919
"Diet in Tuberculosis," 1922
"Food and Food Values," 1922
"Some Applications of our Newer Knowledge of Nutrition," 1922
"How to Meet the Problem of the Delicate Child," 1923
*"Wise Buying of Food," 1923
*"The High Cost of Growing," 1924
"Maintenance Values for the Proteins of Milk, Meat, Bread and Milk, and Soy Bean Curd," 1925
"A Comparison of the Basal Metabolism of Normal Women with Present Prediction Standards," 1925

**Popular or semipopular*
†*Cited as books by the Library of Congress, Washington, D.C.*

Table 7.1—*Continued*

*"Food After Forty," 1925
"The Influence of Prolonged Administration of Egg Upon the Hemoglobin Content of Children's Blood," 1926
"Some Factors Influencing the Basal Metabolism of Children," 1926
*"Is the Study of Nutrition Worth While?" 1926
"Iron in the Diet of Normal Children," 1927
"What Metabolic Research Has Taught in Nutrition of Children," 1927
"A Health Experiment in Harlem," 1927
*"What Sweets Shall Children Have?" 1927
†"Choosing Food for Health," *Handbook on Positive Health,* 1928
"Visualizing Food Values," 1928
*"What Are Green Vegetables?" 1928
*"Foods That Go Together," 1928
*"The Baby's Automobile Kit," 1928
*"What About Dried Fruits?" 1928
"What Place Have Aluminum, Copper, Manganese, and Zinc in Normal Nutrition?" 1929
*"Do You Agree with Your Food?" 1929
*"When My Boy Goes to College, Who Will Feed Him?" 1929
"Functions of Vitamins in Normal Nutrition," 1930
"The Nutritional Significance of Some Mineral Elements Occurring as Traces in the Animal Body," 1932
"University Teaching of Nutrition and Dietetics in the United States," 1935
"Racial Food Habits in Relation to Health," 1937
"A Review of Investigations on the Nutritive Value of Eggs," 1938
*"Protective Foods," 1940
*"Nutrition of Man," 1940

**Popular or semipopular*
†Cited as books by the Library of Congress, Washington, D.C.

Feeding the Family Published in 1916, *Feeding the Family* made such an important contribution to the education of the public that it well deserves special consideration. It was one of the most popular of Rose's publications, not only with the homemaker and others not technically trained who desired help in their choice and use of food but also with the professional in nutrition because it was a new kind of book, a book in which calories, protein, fats, and minerals (vitamins were only beginning to be studied) became foods for men, women, and children and menus for the family.

In the preface, Rose stated:

> While many things contribute to health—sleep, fresh air, and exercise, for instance—the foremost consideration is food. This is recognized today as never before, and those who regard their own welfare and desire to give their children the best possible equipment for the stress of modern life are asking how to choose food wisely. So many kinds of food are displayed in our markets, and so many placards offer warning or advice about what to eat, that a guidebook to good nutrition would seem essential for the twentieth century family. The purpose of the author has been to provide such a little book for the numerous housewives who prepare something like a thousand meals a year for their families and who wish to know how the science of nutrition can be made to function most successfully in their daily lives.[16]

One wonders what Rose would think about today's food markets.

Chapters in the book considered the significance of food; care of the digestive system; food for the adult man, for the adult woman, for the baby, for the two-year-old child, for children three and four years old, for children five to seven years old, for children eight to twelve years old, food in adolescence and youth and food after fifty; food for the family group with regard to menus, cost of food, and food plans and dietaries; and, finally, food for the sick and convalescent.

Over 60,000 copies of this edition were printed. The book was later revised three times. In all, over 150,000 copies of *Feeding the Family* were printed. In the preface of later editions, Rose stated:

> In the years which have elapsed since the first appearance of this book, there has been an increasing application of our knowledge of the importance of a carefully chosen diet for child development and the maintenance of vigor in the adult. This has come about through the accumulation of evidence that growth is directly influenced by food and that a diet which may be adequate for the growth of the young to normal maturity may not be entirely satisfactory for the mother during the periods in which the child is directly dependent upon her for its nourishment. Both before and after birth mineral elements and vitamins greatly affect the development of the child and the vigor of his tissues. To a considerable degree they influence the ability of the mother to furnish milk adequate for growth during the critical first year.

> As a result of such knowledge we have increased emphasis upon the daily use of rich sources of vitamins A and D, such as egg yolk and cod liver oil, and of vitamins B and C, such as orange juice and tomato juice or their equivalents, at all times when growth is involved. Also we have now cognizance of the fact that an adult as well as a growing child will profit by a diet which is of better quality than demanded for mere maintenance; and the hope that by more liberal use of milk and green vegetables we may improve the health and increase the resistance of all the members of the family to bacterial infections of certain sorts which, while not always leading to specific diseases, do decrease the vigor of the tissues and often pave the way for more serious troubles.[17]

CONTACTS WITH PEOPLE

Mary Swartz Rose received many letters requesting her opinion and advice on foods and nutrition, which she answered in a forthright manner, even though the response might not have been what was expected. For example, inquiry regarding her opinion of the material in a booklet entitled *Foods in Relation to Health* for households, brought forth:

> One phrase bothers me a little—"Eat what you want after you have eaten what you should." It rather implies that you will not like what you should eat, doesn't it? It is better said at the bottom of page 3. Only I would like: "Eat your protective foods first," other things you like can be added if you can afford them.[18]

She always took time from her already crowded schedule to reply scientifically and with assurance to housewives and other individuals. In answering a question about using an aluminum kettle—"Don't you think acid food especially should not be cooked in this type of utensil?"—she wrote:

> With regard to aluminum cooking utensils, I can assure you that they present no problem whatever. Aluminum is not absorbed through the alimentary tract and the average daily diet contains more aluminum than would be obtained from cooking in aluminum vessels. This matter has been very thoroughly investigated and there is a large amount of experimental data.[19]

Mary Swartz Rose was very interested in people working with the public on nutrition problems. In many cases she encouraged them to continue with their programs even though they may have been considering further study at the time. She believed "the way to improve nutrition is to work on a one-to-one basis, starting with where the person is now."[20]

Nutrition has become a science to live by—MSR

chapter eight IN INTERNATIONAL AND NATIONAL ORGANIZATIONS

ACTIVITIES AND HONORS

Mary Swartz Rose taught at Teachers College, Columbia University for thirty-one years. She conducted research in nutrition that made her well known and highly respected among scientists. She developed principles related to nutrition problems that were adopted in the United States and throughout the world. In addition to all this, she participated in the programs and activities of many international and national organizations, sometimes as a member of an advisory or work committee, sometimes as a speaker, sometimes as an officer within the society, but always as one who took an active part in what was being done or to be done. She did not dwell on the past and on what might have been. She had an interest in history and a fine grasp of historical events. She used these as stepping-stones to the future and as guides to be applied in the prevention of pitfalls.

Mary Swartz Rose gave distinguished service to many organizations and received many honors and awards. Internationally, she served as a member of the Technical Commission on Nutrition of the Health Organization of the League of Nations and attended its meetings in London in 1935 and 1937 and in Geneva in 1936. There were two other members from the United States—W. Henry Sebrell, Jr., director of the National Institutes of Health, Washington, D.C., and E. V. McCollum, professor of biochemistry, Johns Hopkins University. Rose described the origin of the Technical Commission in an address:

> Many persons are keenly aware of the activities of the League of Nations in the field of international diplomacy, but perhaps even more significant for the permanent welfare of the world are the movements sponsored by the League which bring into friendly cooperation those who have the health of the people as their major aim. Such is the work of the Health Organization of the League. This work has many aspects; at present our concern is with one only—activities in the field of nutrition. . . .
>
> In 1934, having tended to make a general report on the nutritional status of the peoples of Western Europe and the United States, the League delegated Dr. W. R. Aykroyd and Dr. Et. Burnet to visit various countries and study the situation at first hand. Their observations are embodied in a pamphlet, "Nutrition and Public Health" which presents admirably some of the studies leading to the recognition that in most, if not all countries, the health of the people is possible of great improvement through better diet. This report also reviews the various means by which some of the countries are endeavoring to safeguard and educate the people with regard to food. The report makes very clear the very modern point of view that health requirements are not necessarily met when people seem to have enough to eat, and cites many instances where improvement has followed simple changes in diet. . . .
>
> The Burnet and Aykroyd report made such a profound impression that at the September, 1935, assembly in Geneva, twelve governments requested that nutrition problems be placed on the agenda of the next assembly. In due season such a committee was appointed, including agricultural, economic and health experts to submit a report to the assembly in September, 1936. This committee, under the Chairmanship of Lord Astor, is now known as the Mixed Committee.
>
> In order to provide a physiological basis for the Mixed Committee, a special Commission of Nutrition Experts was called to London in November, 1935 to define more clearly the nutritional needs of human beings. . . . The revised report . . . endorses a new principle in world nutrition—i.e., to secure for all peoples in the areas considered a diet which will not merely sustain life, but promote optimum health. Such a diet is one capable of improving the condition of those who seem to be enjoying ordinary health. This means a new standard of well-being—"only the excellent child is a normal one."[1]

The Technical Commission report published in 1936, which Rose considered significant, ended with a list of ten proposals that the commission felt needed further investigation. These are given below, as arranged in order of priority:

- Assessment of the state of nutrition in children and adolescents
- Nutritive food requirements during the first year of life
- Minimum vitamin and mineral requirements
- Minimum fat requirements
- The nutritive and "supplementary" values of the different protein-containing foods to determine to what extent and in what forms animal protein is necessary for growth and health
- The relative nutritive value of different cereals according to the degree of milling
- The extent to which the increasing consumption of sugar is detrimental to health
- Influence of climate on food requirements
- The extent to which diets in common use fall below the standards recommended in this report
- The optimum amounts of milk required at different ages.[2]

Over forty years later, and we have not answered many of these proposals!

Rose stated in an address that the aims of the Mixed Committee were:

- The pursuit and support of progress in nutrition
- Simplification and dissemination of the results of scientific research
- The raising to the level of an indisputable social principle, the collective obligation to provide mothers, infants, children, and poor persons with an indispensable nutrition minimum
- The creation in all countries of a definite nutrition policy
- The creation of organizations to give life to this policy.[3]

And over forty years later, we have not reached these aims.

The report was a best seller, however, and even though the league did not continue as a political organization, the work in food and agriculture survived and probably set the plan for subsequent international efforts in nutrition.

Mary Swartz Rose found the meetings of the Technical Commission very interesting. She played an active part in the work of the commission and in the preparation of its reports. She influenced the commission's recommendations, particularly with regard to milk requirements. When she returned from the meeting in Geneva, she told of the difficulty in getting a quart of milk into the child's dietary requirements. The French delegate "didn't think a child's small stomach would take a quart of milk." Rose said that she could not have returned to the United States if she had not been able to accomplish this.[4] In response to a question from New Zealand regarding the recommendation, she wrote:

> It is hard to put in the brief compass of a letter the evidence which has led to the recommendation of a quart of milk a day in the diet of the growing child and the pregnant and lactating woman. In this country, the same recommendation is extended to adults who wish to safeguard their diets in the easiest possible way.

Then she proceeded to convincingly cite Dr. McCollum, her own "Foundations of Nutrition," Sherman's "Food Products," and Dr. Lydia J. Roberts' study.[5]

It is regrettable that Mary Swartz Rose did not enjoy the sea voyages to these meetings. As she wrote to a friend regarding Dr. McCollum's suggestion that she sail on the same ship with him and Dr. Sebrell, "It would make me so sad (or mad) to be lying below and 'those boys' having a jolly time above!"[6]

Mary Swartz Rose was active in several important national groups (table 8.1). She served as a member of the Council on Foods and Nutrition of the American Medical Association for many years. At the request of the council she reviewed the available evidence on the nutritive value of quick-frozen foods and prepared a report for publication.[7] Partly on the basis of this report, the council voted to give consideration to quick-frozen vegetables and fruits with a view to including them in their list of accepted foods.

Following her death, the council authorized publication of this statement:

> Mrs. Rose was one of the outstanding teachers of her time. Through her classes at Teachers College she came to exert a wide influence on the development of nutrition and the teaching of this science in many institutions throughout the country. . . . She brought her talents as a writer effectively to bear on the problem of education of the general public in matters concerning foods and nutrition. In the midst of these

> many activities she also proved that she could be a productive scholar adding to the sum total of scientific knowledge in this field. . . . Because of her unusual qualities, she was also called on to render important public services. . . .
>
> From this brief statement it is evident why Dr. Rose should have been elected to membership in the Council on Foods. To the Council's deliberations she brought a wide experience that touched not merely the academic sphere of interest but the general public welfare and education of both the public and food industry, matters of great importance in relation to the work which the Council was established to perform. These counsels were effectively rendered because they came from one also endowed with much personal charm.[8]

Now, when the American Institute of Nutrition has been celebrating its fiftieth anniversary, it is fitting to recall Mary Swartz Rose's role in this important national organization. As already mentioned, she was the only woman in the group of eleven founders. She became its fifth president, the first woman to hold that office. At the annual meeting held in Baltimore, March 30, 1938, over which she presided, several

TABLE 8.1 Memberships in National Organizations

American Association for the Advancement of Science, member 1908, and fellow, 1926
American Child Health Association
American Dietetic Association
American Home Economics Association
American Institute of Nutrition, founder, 1928
American Physiological Society
American Public Health Association, fellow, 1922
American Society of Biological Chemists
Council on Foods and Nutrition of American Medical Association
Harvey Society
National Child Health Council
National Education Association
Omicron Nu
Sigma Xi
Society for Biological Chemists
Society of Experimental Biology and Medicine

scientific sessions and group meetings were held. The dinner that evening in honor of Russell H. Chittenden, professor emeritus of Yale University, was attended by three hundred members and their friends. One of the members said of Mary Swartz Rose:

> It seems to me that her conduct of the American Institute was an outstanding success and her talk at the Institute banquet was one of the most interesting and human discussions we have ever had. . . . she made up some of the cleverest charts regarding each of the former council members. . . . at the meeting Mrs. Rose was at her best.[9]

Her further activities in this organization included service for many years as a member of the editorial board of *The Journal of Nutrition* (fig. 8.1).

On Mary Swartz Rose's sixty-fifth birthday she was given the Award of Distinction by the Associated Grocery Manufacturers of America "in recognition of her contributions to the science of nutrition, the great part she has played in the dissemination of scientific information concerning foods, and her authorship in this field, and her outstanding career as a teacher of others who teach nutrition."[10] (Table 8.2 lists honors and distinguished service.) At the ceremonies, it was said that the award that year had a double distinction. First, the presentation address was made by Henry C. Sherman who had received the award previously and second, it was the first time the award was made to a woman (fig. 8.2). In his remarks, Sherman said of Mary Swartz Rose:

> As scientist, as teacher, as nutrition publicist, she is rendering her generation a service so fundamental and so far-reaching in this formative period of her chosen profession that it is built into the very fabric of a new and permanent phase of human progress where it will continue to serve all of the generations who are to come.
>
> It is a truism and an understatement to speak of her worldwide influence—worldwide, yes, surely, and a deep and a high influence, too.[11]

In accepting the award, Rose said:

> It is with great humility that I accept this honor which you have so graciously accorded me. The few small steps which one worker can take toward ultimate truth are rewarding to the person that makes them, out

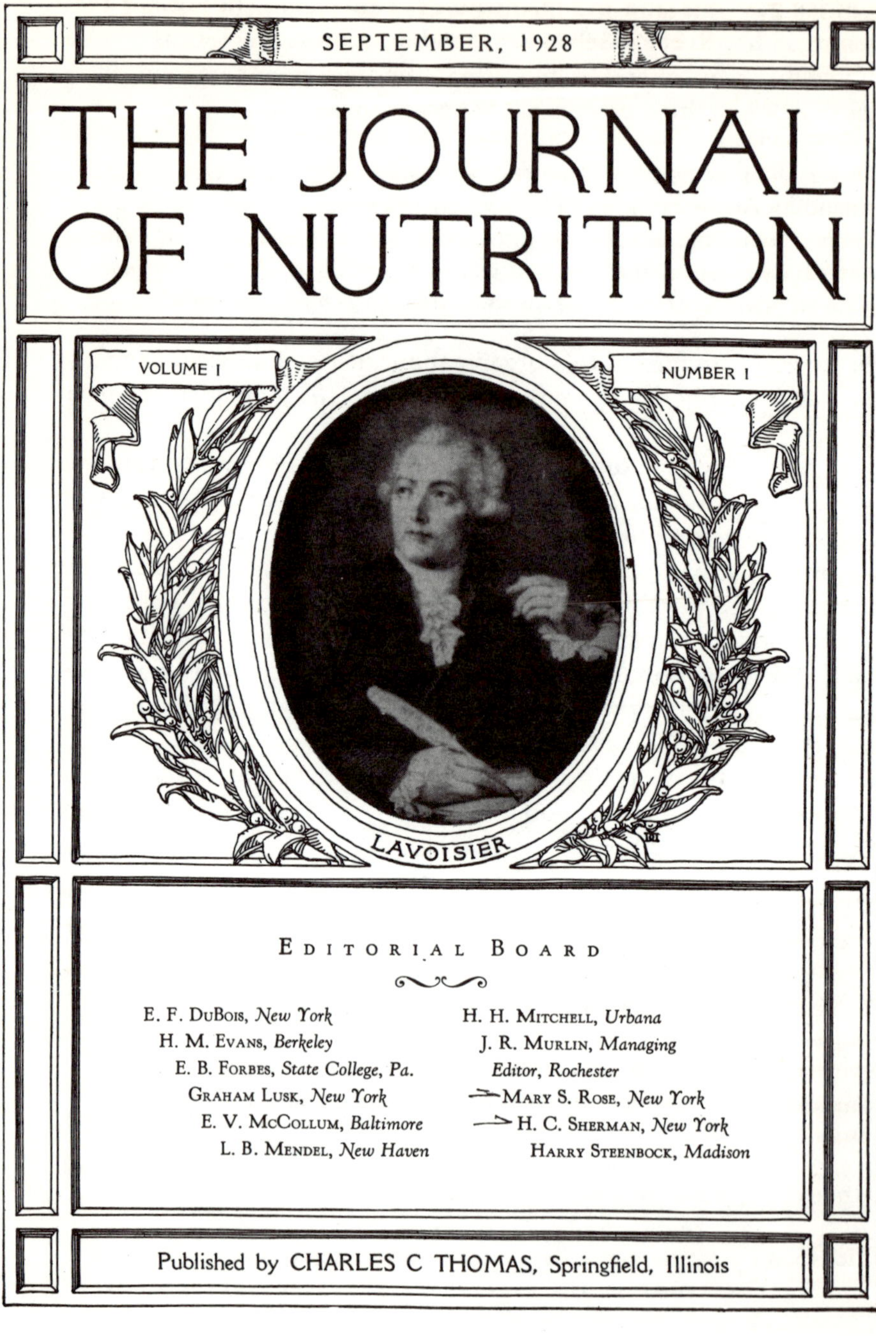
SEPTEMBER, 1928

THE JOURNAL OF NUTRITION

VOLUME I

NUMBER I

LAVOISIER

EDITORIAL BOARD

E. F. DuBois, *New York*
H. M. Evans, *Berkeley*
E. B. Forbes, *State College, Pa.*
Graham Lusk, *New York*
E. V. McCollum, *Baltimore*
L. B. Mendel, *New Haven*
H. H. Mitchell, *Urbana*
J. R. Murlin, *Managing Editor, Rochester*
Mary S. Rose, *New York*
H. C. Sherman, *New York*
Harry Steenbock, *Madison*

Published by CHARLES C THOMAS, Springfield, Illinois

Fig. 8.1 The Journal of Nutrition, *vol. I, no. 1*

TABLE 8.2 Honors and Distinguished Service, with Date of Recognition

Wooster High School, valedictorian, 1892

Teachers College, Columbia University, traveling fellow, 1907

Sigma Xi, first woman elected to Yale University chapter, 1909

Connecticut Academy of Arts and Sciences, member, 1909

Bureau of Food Conservation, New York State Food Commission and Federal Food Board, deputy director, 1918

American Institute of Nutrition, member of Board of Directors, 1928; founder, 1928; vice-president, 1936; first woman president, 1937

Journal of Nutrition, member of Editorial Board, 1928

White House Conference on Child Health, member of Committee on Growth and Development, 1931

Who's Who in American Education, listed, 1931

American Medical Association, member of Committee on Foods and Nutrition, 1933

Women's Medical Journal, member of Editorial Committee, 1934

Who's Who among North American Authors, listed, 1933

Health Organization of the League of Nations, member of Technical Commission on Nutrition, 1935

One of twelve career women honored in celebration of Business Woman's Week, New York City, 1935

Chosen by international quarterly *Nutrition Abstracts and Reviews* to write a comprehensive account and interpretation of the college and university teaching of nutrition and dietetics in the United States, 1935

Honored at a dinner in celebration of her 25th anniversary (1934) at Teachers College; her portrait by Ivan Olinsky was presented to the college by her former students, 1936

The New York Herald Tribune, a member of advisory staff, 1936

American Men of Science, listed, 1938

Council of National Defense, advisor on nutrition, 1940

National Research Council, consultant to Committee on Food and Nutrition, 1940

First woman to receive the annual award of distinction of the Associated Grocery Manufacturers of America, 1940

Emeritus Professor, 1940

American Dietetic Association, honorary member, 1940

Omicron Nu, honorary member, 1940

Who's Who in America, 1940

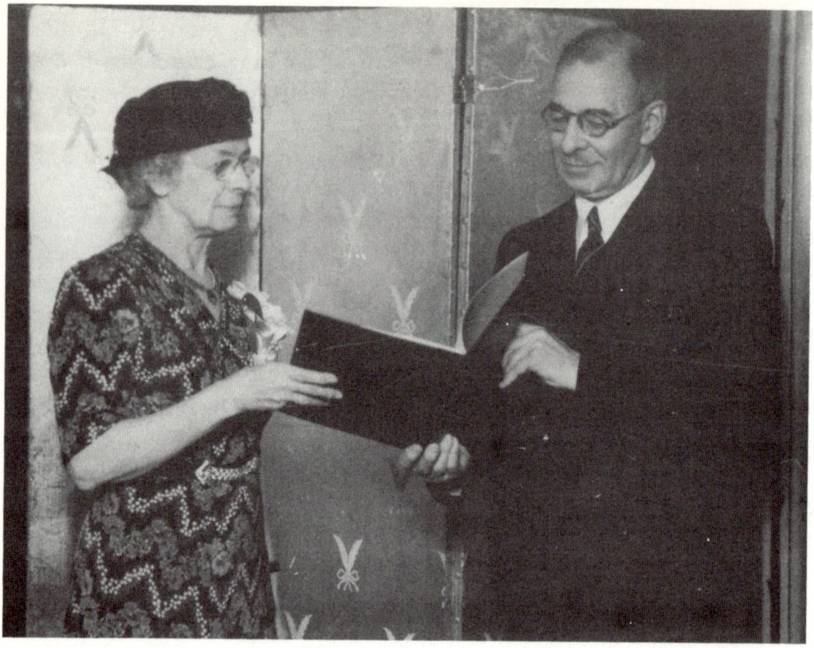

Fig. 8.2 Henry C. Sherman presents the Associated Grocery Manufacturers of America Award to Mary Swartz Rose, October 31, 1939

> of all proportion to their contribution to the sum of knowledge. Their maker needs no other reward. But for the sake of my great teachers, Sherman and Mendel, my colleagues who have stood by me through thick and thin, and the institution which has given me opportunity to labor in the cause of science, I thank you for this award.
>
> It is significant because it symbolizes the faith in science of a great organization engaged in work of the most fundamental importance for human welfare—the nation's food.

The last great honor bestowed upon Mary Swartz Rose during her lifetime was an honorary membership in the American Dietetic Association in 1940 in appreciation of her distinguished contribution to nutrition, an occasion noted in a publication of the association:

> It has been the custom of this Association to grant, from time to time, honorary membership to a select few whose works and precepts have served to lead and encourage us through the years.
>
> To this honored group, another name is to be added—that of a woman known to all here, and to thousands throughout the far corners

of the United States and other lands where the science of nutrition, largely by her efforts, has become an almost magic force for human betterment. A veritable human dynamo, she has activated an army of zealous workers who have gone out from that great university, Columbia, and with almost religious fervor, have spread far and wide the gospel of good nutrition.

In keeping with her womanly devotion to human needs, her interests have centered mainly on children, in whom lies our hope for a better world—physically, mentally and morally. Hers has been an almost saintly devotion to their cause. And her works, above all others, I believe, have been the means whereby thousands of children may now reach their adult years, strong in body, happy and eager for life's work and play.

But one cannot measure her worth by this alone, forceful though it be. For Mary Swartz Rose, scientist, and beloved teacher of thousands of students, will always be enshrined in their hearts—a happy, vivid, warm, and spiritual force that makes us all believe in the innate goodness of the human race, despite what is happening today. She has stood out, through the years, like an unwavering beacon, lighting our way, cheering our hearts—to us, an immortal.[12]

POSTHUMOUS HONORS

In 1942, the year after her death, the Greater New York Dietetic Association established the Mary Swartz Rose Memorial Lecture. Each year a distinguished scientist has been selected to give this lecture in her honor in New York City.

Eight years after her death, with funds from the Nutrition Foundation, the American Dietetic Association set up a fellowship named in her honor to perpetuate her ideals of professional achievement. Clara Mae Taylor presented the first fellowship in 1949.[13]

In 1957 a fellowship honoring Mary Swartz Rose was established at Teachers College by her former associates and by gifts from the alumni. This fellowship is awarded to students in the field of nutrition education.

ADDRESSES

Rose interpreted the findings of nutrition research through her speeches to many professional and scholarly organizations. She desired that the truths of the science be applied to daily living in order that healthful nutrition practices be followed.

In 1912 she gave her first address outside the classroom to the New York Agricultural Society on the topic of "homemakers' problems." She opened her address with:

> When . . . asked . . . if I would come here to speak to you, I was in the city of Washington, and I thought that the experience I was having there bore directly on the housewife's problem. I found that wherever I went, following directions as well as I could, I usually had to walk five or six blocks when they told me the car went past the door. I found that I paid about twice as much for meals as anyone else because I did not know the best places to go; and I found that here, there, and everywhere I was paying in time and money and energy the price of ignorance. Now it seems to me that is what the housewife is doing all the time when she tries to feed her family without a knowledge of food values.[14]

Then she spoke of the foods needed by the family, relating their costs to their nutritive values.

Over the years she addressed national as well as state and local organizations. When she wished to deliver a particular message to several different groups of people, people with varying interests and backgrounds, she sometimes used the same speech outline. And sometimes she was requested to repeat a particular address to another audience. She always, however, adapted a repeated address to the particular situation and group. Frequently she would revise the speech once again for publication in an appropriate journal so that a still larger audience could be reached (table 8.3).

It is not known how many addresses she made during her professional life: she was a prized public speaker and she delivered many addresses. Among her private papers, outlines were found for the following unpublished addresses:

"Nutrition Activities of the League of Nations," 1936
"The Nutrition of the School Child," 1936
"Nutrition and the 20th Century Child," 1937
"Looking Forward in Health," 1938
"Nutrition—A Means to Better Health," 1938
"Consumer Standards for Food Expenditures," 1939
"Recent Findings in Nutrition Related to Child Development," 1939
"New Ways of Looking at Old Foods," 1940
"World Movements in Nutrition," 1940

TABLE 8.3 Published Addresses, with Date of Publication and Group Addressed

"The Question of Child Feeding," 1919, Second Annual Convention of the American Dietetic Association

"Recent Developments in Child Feeding," 1920, Home Economics Conference of the Michigan Agricultural College

"Child Nutrition and Diet," 1923, Fifth Annual Meeting of the American Dietetic Association

"What Is Progress in Nutrition?" 1925, 17th Annual Meeting of the American Home Economics Association

"Ten Years of Vitamin Research," 1926, Vocational Home Economics Teachers State Meeting

"Old and New Emphasis in the Teaching of Nutrition," 1930, Food and Nutrition Section, American Home Economics Association

"Belief in Magic," 1932, Annual Dinner of American Dietetic Association

"Our Children and Their Nutrition Needs," 1932, American Red Cross Society

"Nutrition in the Life of the Growing Child," 1934, Food and Nutrition Division, American Home Economics Association, New York City

"Nutrition and Health of the School Child," 1939, General Session of American Dietetic Association

At her last public appearance, November 14, 1940, she spoke on "World Movements in Nutrition" to the New Jersey Dietetic Association. She had given this speech previously, with modifications, at Wellesley College, at Rhode Island State College, to teachers of homemaking of the New York City schools and to the students in the College of Physicians and Surgeons, Columbia University. In the address, she emphasized the conquest of science and nutrition in different countries. In closing she stated:

> The advance of science opens to us the opportunity of raising the standard of living to a higher level than it has ever attained in the history of mankind. And an adequate diet is certainly the most important element in the standard of living. Malnutrition is like an iceberg; its greatest mass and its greatest danger lie beneath the surface. On the other hand, greater benefits than the mere absence of disease or nutritional deficiency result from an abundance of these foods in the diet

which insure plenty of minerals and vitamins—*the protective foods*—milk, green vegetables, whole grains and fruits.

If all the people were to have diets as adequate as are enjoyed by many in the higher income levels, more farm land would have to be put into production. If milk consumption were at the level best suited to maintaining an adequate diet, we should need a million and a half more cows. There would have to be an expansion of production of almost every food except wheat, and if every person were to receive a full ration of calories, it is doubtful whether there would be any occasion to curtail wheat. The success of a policy to improve nutrition depends upon many factors—agriculture, transportation, tariff barriers, exchange restrictions, national security, and armament policy as well as on the efforts of those specifically interested in the public health. We do not know yet how to achieve the "marriage of agriculture and public health" but we recognize it as the great social obligation of our times.[15]

Recent discussions of the need for a national food policy have taken place in professional associations and government agencies, even in the Senate of the United States, and still we do not have a national food policy.

Below are some quotations from Rose's published addresses expressing her views:

We ought to have such standards of health as would make us uncomfortable to be out of health, just as we feel uncomfortable if our clothes are out of fashion. . . . Not survival of the fittest . . . but all surviving and fit, the true test of a vigorous, civilized race.[16]

We are investing enormous sums in education and are destined to invest very much more. Without a long, efficient life, how can this education upon which the hope of our country is staked give us an adequate return on our investment?[17]

The great task in education is how to live so as to realize one's highest possibilities. . . . School feeding must be educational to have lasting value.[18]

In childhood, the habits of health must be formed.[19]

This (2–6 years) is the most critical period in the formation of good eating habits, a time demanding constant education in eating. . . . Training in table manners, in eating what is set before one, in dining rather than feeding, are important parts of making a child a good social being, though they are less important than the training in what is good food and how to eat it.[20]

> There are many interested in . . . "the humanizing of knowledge" but let us pray for a little more knowledge before the humanizing is begun! . . . When we have finally had "recourse to . . . all the sciences which bear, directly or indirectly, on the great processes of eating and digestion," . . . we must bring these scattered contributions together and from contemplation of all their implications construct practical programs, fitted to each locality, and so far as possible, to each individual. We must not forget the limitations imposed by climate, by season, by human labor, by the contents of pocket books. We must study milk and eggs and spinach and oatmeal—all common foods—and see that our own likes or dislikes or social customs do not influence our conclusions as to their intrinsic merits.[21]

Malnutrition is a term used very broadly for all sorts of divergences from the normal in physical and mental vigor, but in the growing organism its most common manifestations are interference with growth and the lack of resistance to disease.[22]

Our chances of good nutrition are immensely increased when we know how to choose—MSR

chapter nine STUDENTS OF ROSE

Former nutrition students of Teachers College are found in schools and colleges, in local, state, national and international government agencies, and in service organizations throughout the United States and foreign lands.

When discussing the aims of Teachers College in 1909, President Nicholas Murray Butler made the following remarks:

> It has steadily pursued the path marked out for it in the beginning, of treating education as a unit resting on a philosophic foundation. . . . The work of Teachers College is the model upon which reformers in education all over the world shape their proposals. It is constantly visited by educators and educationists of rank and distinction from all parts of the world. Its graduates are to be found in schools and colleges of every class and every type in foreign lands, as well as in each of the United States.[1]

Then in 1915, the aims of the nutrition program at Teachers College were recorded as:

> The study of nutrition is not only an interesting academic pursuit, touching clinical, physiological, and bacteriological science on the one hand and psychology, economics, and sociology on the other, but is also of great practical importance for the welfare of the human race. A double obligation therefore rests with this department to give thorough training in the fundamental principles of the subject, and to dissemi-

nate freely the facts of nutrition in such form as will best reach the public.[2]

Approximately 11,000 students were enrolled in Mary Swartz Rose's classes over the years; some were majors in nutrition, others were from the chemistry department at Columbia, and from related fields of home economics, nursing, science education, and other areas with an interest in nutrition (fig. 9.1). Over twenty-five graduate nutrition students of Rose served as assistants in the department (table 9.1).

Many of the students in Mary Swartz Rose's classes attended the summer sessions at Teachers College. During the summers of 1928 and 1940 Rose was a visiting professor at Oregon State College, in 1936 at Iowa State College, and in 1940 at Florida State College. She traveled abroad with her husband and son in 1929, 1932, and 1935. Grace MacLeod was in charge of the summer sessions at Teachers College when Rose was absent.

For a period Teachers College also offered extension courses. There was a demand for nutrition courses from public school teachers that took Mary Swartz Rose to a number of areas outside New York City.

TABLE 9.1 Graduate Student Assistants, Teaching and/or Research, 1913–40

Helene Pope	Gertrude Christie
Ada Field	Gertrude Dinsmore
Irma Latzer	Helen Taylor
Gertrude Mudge	Flora Edmonds
Martha Dresslar	Catherine Newton
Hannah Honewell	Esther Funnell (Phipard)
Margaret Fedde	Adeline Missal
Margaret Sandels	Bertlyn Bosley
Elda Robb	Ruth Pike
Ella McCollum (Vahlteich)	Eloise Cofer
Ruth Strang	Katherine Nugent
Harriet Stone	Emma Gardner
Gertrude Preischer	Orrea F. Pye
Clara Mae Taylor	

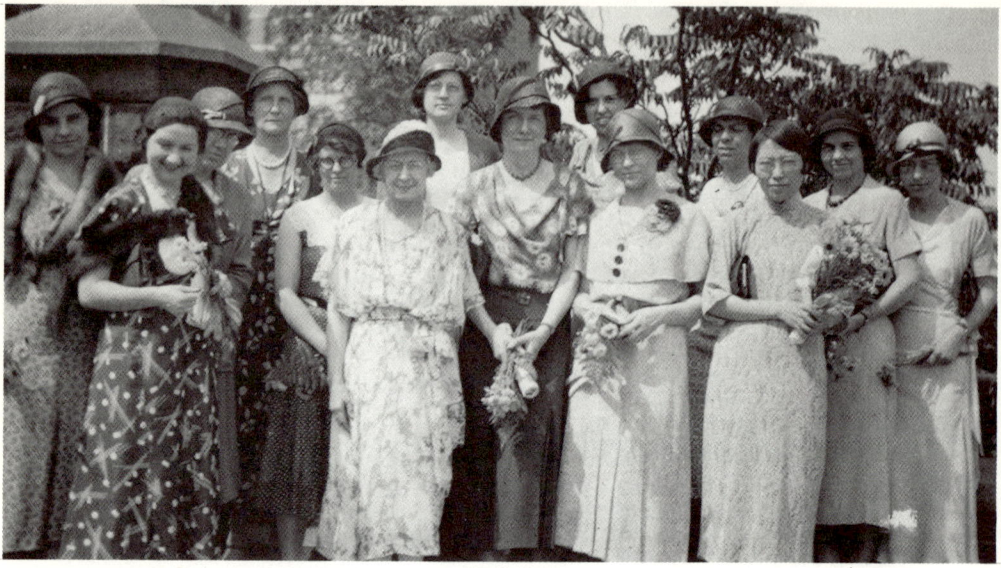

Fig. 9.1 Following a luncheon given by Mary Swartz Rose to honor the Ph.D. candidates Kung, Potgieter, and Robb—left to right: *Clara Mae Taylor, Charlotte Herter, Professor MacLeod, Helen Hubbell, Dorothy Williams, Professor Rose, Imogene Manning, Martha Potgieter, Marie O'Donahoe, Elda Robb, Adeline Missal, Lan-Chen Kung, Esther Funnell (Phipard), Miss Brown*

Clara Mae Taylor usually taught these courses with Rose and recalls a very cold, snowy, and icy day when they journeyed out to Hempstead, Long Island. Rose had had an operation on her foot and was walking with crutches, but insisted on taking the class because "it was her turn" even though Taylor offered to do so.[3]

Mary McCormick, who had been appointed instructor in the nutrition program in 1911, has reported:

> In those early years when lectures were the almost exclusive method of teaching in most college classrooms, Mrs. Rose was successfully using discussion as one of her teaching techniques. She led discussion brilliantly. Penetrating questions, quick evaluation of student responses, and the ability to use student experiences in building up and integrating group thinking made her a masterly teacher. In fact, she had few equals.
>
> The seminar for graduate students met weekly from 4:00 to 6:00 P.M.

> when the students were tired from their day's work. Their response to the long papers (reports on recent research in the various scientific journals) was often dispirited. Mrs. Rose originated the plan of having each report condensed to *one sheet,* which the department had mimeographed and distributed to the students when the longer report was presented. The result was electrifying in stimulating alertness, interest, and discussion. During all class periods, but especially during the seminar, one of Mrs. Rose's dominant aims was that of helping the students to base their judgments on experimental evidence and not on opinions, and at the same time developing in those students confidence in themselves, as exponents and proponents of the scientific facts already established. She recognized these women as future leaders, as indeed many of them became.[4]

Henry C. Sherman was a regular participant in the nutrition seminars at Teachers College until he retired from Columbia University. He was a good listener and waited to be sure whether someone wanted his opinion or was trying to inform him. He would chuckle and say "They didn't want my advice, they wanted to tell me." Rose was very strict about the seminars and quickly learned to be critical of the students' reports. Sherman acted as a moderator, saying "Now don't you think . . ." Mary Swartz Rose was very conscious of people and aware of human needs. She was compassionate and considerate of the students and made arrangements for their creature comforts, such as having tea before the seminars.

Her colleagues paid tribute to Rose's contributions to education. Her dean, James Earl Russell, in praising her accomplishments as a teacher, said:

> She . . . had no selfish interest which ever stood between her and her students. . . . Few women in her time were her superior in scholarly attainment, teaching ability, and service in the public welfare. Her life was an honor to our profession.[5]

Grace MacLeod, her coteacher for many years, said of her teaching:

> She was clear, incisive, painstaking, stimulating. . . . She counted no amount of time and care too great to spend in preparation and planning for her classes if it promised better results for the student, whether in the elementary grades or in the most advanced college work.[6]

Henry C. Sherman, her former teacher and later associate, wrote:

> Mrs. Rose . . . would say that her best discoveries are the students who have gone from her training into positions of leadership.[7]

When Mary Swartz Rose had completed twenty-five years of teaching, her students wished to mark the anniversary in a way that would express their appreciation to her and to Teachers College. They arranged for her portrait to be painted by Ivan Olinsky and presented it to the college at a dinner held in her honor at the Women's Faculty Club of Columbia University, October 19, 1936. It was a festive occasion with her husband, academic friends, and others present. Grace MacLeod represented the students (see Appendix B, page 166) and Mary de Garmo Bryan, professor of Institutional Management at Teachers College, was toastmistress.

It was the intention of the authors to contact Rose's former students regarding her influence on them and on their life work. In reviewing archival materials, however, we found that in 1941 following Mary Swartz Rose's death questionnaires had been sent to her former students requesting just this information. Clyde B. Schuman, who sent the questionnaires, was a former student herself and desired to write about Mary Swartz Rose as a scientist and teacher for her doctoral thesis at New York University. In the spring of 1940 Mary Swartz Rose had given permission to Schuman to send the questionnaires and had reviewed a tentative copy of the questionnaire during that summer.

Questionnaires were sent to over 3,200 former students in the United States and other countries, approximately 700 who had majored in nutrition, 1,000 in home economics, and 1,500 who had majored in fields other than nutrition or home economics. About 40 percent of the mailing was returned as undeliverable at the given address, but replies were received from over two hundred students. We are indebted to Clyde B. Schuman for recording verbatim their responses in her doctoral thesis.[8] The following statements are taken from her thesis:

> Her classes were crowded with interested students. She possessed to a remarkable degree the ability to "put across" the subject matter; rather, it might be more nearly correct to say that she guided, while the subject matter "put itself across." She was able, in the course of an evening's

lecture, to cover so much of the field that lay persons came away with an astonishing knowledge of practical nutrition. Yet she could conduct seminars with advanced students in a way that spurred them to even greater efforts. (A student at the Florida summer school)

Mrs. Rose taught at Oregon State College for three weeks in the summer session of 1940. She conducted two courses: "Recent Advances in Nutrition" and "Teaching Problems in Nutrition." The latter course dealt with problems of high school teaching. . . . Mrs. Rose was especially full of vivacity and energy during her stay here. She had a number of ideas not only for teaching that summer, but for the future. She wanted to put them all into practice immediately. She charmed all of her students as well as the staff. She gave two or three extra lectures in the evenings, which were so well attended that many people had to sit on stools or stand in order to hear her. (A professor of foods and nutrition who had been a former student)

She taught us to accept nothing but information that was scientifically sound. She cautioned us, however, to be tolerant always. Her procedures and habits of work both in the laboratory and in the classroom were systematic and she was untiring in her interest and effort. (A former student who was a nutrition consultant for the Georgia State Health Department.)

Dr. Rose was, I believe, a friend to all her students. She was *exacting* in that she wanted things correct, and to her I owe a great deal for this characteristic. In no field are there so many misstatements made as in nutrition. She taught us to be specific, to remember that it wasn't any discredit not to know the answer to every question asked us, but that the discredit came when we didn't look up the information and answer the question to the best of our ability. It was our duty to know where to secure the information we sought. (A head dietitian at a hospital)

As a student of Dr. Rose she gave me something of herself—that something which establishes a warm relationship with the student. . . . She helped me to seek a goal, but to be aware of means; to analyze and on that basis to make decisions. As a leader she helped me to evaluate the situation—to plan the working relationship with people, and to find satisfaction in work well done. She helped me to develop perspective—to be willing to wait for a change—to have the long-time viewpoint. (An assistant supervisor of nutrition in East Harlem Nursing and Health Demonstration)

She did not consider that you knew facts and had information until they were yours in their relationship to practical nutrition problems. . . . I feel that Mrs. Rose's teaching was challenging to the best students in her classes. At the same time she was sympathetic with those who had difficulty in keeping up. She had a keen insight into human nature and was past master at human relationships. (Chief of a university division of home economics)

She deplored the tendency of those who spend their lives in careful research to publish their findings in a form which does not appeal to the laity. She believed that with those who were privileged to know rested the responsibility of passing on the truths of nutrition findings to others. (A community service worker in nutrition)

Mrs. Rose's influence on my teaching has been very great. My position is in a rural school. I am thoroughly familiar with the diet deficiencies of my pupils and some of the resultant diseases. Pellagra has long been a scourge in our section through ignorance of the right way of eating. Although I teach fourth graders, we make vitamin and mineral charts and *eat* the foods that give us the vitamins, minerals and other nutrients needed. The mothers come to me to find out more about vitamins so that they may give their children what "the teacher" talks about. (A teacher from the southern states)

Her own standards were so high you didn't want to fall short of what she expected. I can remember several incidents illustrating this. She had little patience with the slacker, but ever so much with those who were willing to work. She couldn't tolerate sloppiness or carelessness. (A teacher)

She was the most inspiring teacher I ever had and by that I mean that she stimulated all to their finest and best mental endeavors. Her own logical and penetrating mind led her students into satisfying habits of thought and work. No minute in her classes was ever dull or even ordinary. (A teacher)

Dr. Rose's succinctly stated principles have been my principles and teaching guide-post for many years. An estimate of the influence which Dr. Rose has had upon me would call for a measuring of her indirect influence on my 850 students a week, my family, and my summer campers. (A teacher)

She had an earthy sort of practicalness that always delighted me and made what she taught stick.

Her extended travel and wide reading gave her a balance, a fresh approach at all times. She was skilled with her hands. . . . She practiced her theories. Her superb mental equipment almost dazed one, but warmth of heart and sympathy put one at ease.

I remember her sincere *modesty* in her estimate of her own accomplishments, and her keen *sense of humor* when she thought praise out of proportion. There was always an honest enjoyment of national and international recognition, and never, as is too often the case, a pseudo self-depreciation. She was possessed of a rare integrity of mind and personality.

She left a feeling of warmth and friendliness that remained long after the classroom work was done; that particular feeling that testified to her neverending interest in her students.

Mary Swartz Rose was to me: first a person who was sure of her teachings, because she was scientific and her learning rested upon experimental evidence often repeated; secondly, she believed in breadth of study in life and learning, and, finally, above all she was a woman who lived and helped others live and a humanitarian whose mission was to make learning function.

A number of students came from other countries to study nutrition with Mary Swartz Rose. Schuman sent questionnaires to these former students, some of whom were living under war conditions. There was a gratifying response. The following quotations taken from the responses to the questionnaire and from letters sent voluntarily to Schuman indicate the spread of Rose's influence beyond the United States:

From New Zealand—I was until I retired a few years ago, head of the Home Science Department of Wellington Technical College, and though retired, I am still very actively engaged in doing work for women and girls together with other activities in connection with war work. . . . Though Dr. Rose was unknown to many of my students personally, she lives on as a vivid inspiration through her writings. . . . There was always a thrill amongst us as students when Dr. Rose was to give the lecture.

I feel very strongly that the consideration of nutrition on a scientific basis in New Zealand is due to those teachers who came here from

America more than 25 years ago and who had probably been students or colleagues of the late Dr. Rose. I, as probably one of the very few of any of the pioneer teachers remaining in New Zealand, have watched with interest the growth in our dominion of this important subject to its present stage of wonderful progress and far-reaching effect on the lives and homes of the people, and also in improvement in the management of hospitals, institutions, and commercial concerns. . . .

The privilege of meeting Dr. Rose and having a course in dietetics under her . . . was an experience that gave me inspiration as well as concrete help for carrying on my work in New Zealand.

From Canada—Mrs. Rose was so kind in getting together old graduates and hearing about their work. . . . At one of the conventions several of our students were there. They were delighted to have the opportunity to meet Mrs. Rose. She, of course, in a few happy remarks, called them her grandchildren. . . . I always tell my students about my contact with Mrs. Rose. . . . Our students are stationed in many parts of the British Empire, as well as in the United States. Some have gone to England, South Africa, Australia, also to other places. . . . Mrs. Rose's influence is far-reaching when one considers the students of various students.

From South Africa—I enjoyed Dr. Rose's classes very much and am using some of her methods—or adapting them to use in my physiology and hygiene classes here.

From China—A group of us working in nutrition in North China have been using Dr. Rose's plan of approach in teaching. Two of us have studied with her, and others have caught the enthusiasm from us. . . . On the morning of the 8th of December, 1941, the participation of the Westerner in our work in China ceased. The work of the university on the home campus was closed after the first hour of classes. Since then, folk have said to me, "Isn't it too bad that your work in North China is ended—that it's all stopped?" And I answer: "It hasn't stopped, for all over North China there are children who are being better fed; people who are living more adequate lives, because of the nutrition teaching we have done." In the same way it may be said that Dr. Rose is still teaching; those of us who were her students know that all over the world her work is going on through the work of those whom she taught and who were influenced by her; and will continue through the years in the lives of their students and those with whom they have come in contact.

From Sweden—When I returned to Sweden it was thanks to Mrs. Rose that I got my first position and got started on the road of nutrition in this country. . . . I remember her as a great teacher who gave me inspiration and courage—and also as a good friend who took me into her home and family.

When several former students of Mary Swartz Rose learned that this biography was being written, they wrote to the authors. Their comments regarding Rose as a teacher, made almost forty years after attending her classes, are of interest. One writes:

I remember her as a superb teacher—so perfect that one could hardly think of offering a compliment—but one day when the lesson had been so marvelously presented, I *had* to say something about it, and to my amazement, her appreciation was almost overwhelming.[9]

Another writes:

I remember her as an inspiring teacher and a challenging one whose wishes I had to fulfill. For example: The nutrition teaching in the elementary schools which I did under her direction. The first lesson was a failure but with Mrs. Rose one did not fail again—my next lesson, and all following ones, were a success because she expected it of me.[10]

And another:

One of her "teaching expressions" which I remember and used with marked success in my own work was her frequent reference to the "Red Queen" in *Alice in Wonderland,* who taught that "the way to learn it is to do it."[11]

And:

In the fall of 1915, I registered for courses with Dr. Sherman and with Mary Swartz Rose. The whispered word was then that Dr. Rose was very strict and demanding as a teacher, but interesting and clear. When I came to my first class I first saw this little lady who stood tall and seemed fully in control of herself and the class. The lecture started on the dot of the scheduled hour. One felt guilty if even a few minutes late, as Dr. Rose watched until one reached the appointed place at a long

> table in the lecture room. It gave me a new sense of the importance of punctuality.[12]

From Canada:

> My association with Dr. Rose dates back to 1926 when I went to Columbia University as a student. I was so impressed by Dr. Rose's dedication to spread the importance of good nutrition to persons of all ages that I majored in that field for my master's degree.
>
> Dr. Rose had the endearing quality of treating her students as friends, helping them with personal problems and sharing good times with them in her home. Acting on her advice that a person should stay long enough in one place to improve both the position and the teaching, I stayed thirty-five years at Mount Allison University.[13]

A FAVORITE CLASS

Mary Swartz Rose's director described the growth of the nutrition program at Teachers College in the following way:

> Two things made the department of nutrition grow: first, other departments encouraged their students to take courses, notably the health and physical education course known as Hygiene 101. Mrs. Rose was willing to give a popular course, but unwilling to have a popular course called "Nutrition." When it was proposed to her, she liked the idea, but accepted it under the title of a Hygiene course. It brought her many students and was a success from the beginning. At the same time, Mrs. Rose was more and more attracting advanced graduate students.[14]

The course Hygiene 101 (Nutrition and Health) was her favorite course. She found this course a real challenge and enjoyed it because she was reaching so many students from other areas at the college who would otherwise not know of the importance of nutrition. Rose introduced this course in the academic year 1928–29 and taught it each year until 1940–41. Then, Clara Mae Taylor, who had taught it with Rose for over a decade, continued it under the title Nutrition 101. In this tradition, a non-major course in nutrition is still continued today. Rose kept the five-page outline of notes for her first session in Hygiene 101. Her husband cherished the outline notes and later passed them along to Taylor. The first page reads:

(Hyg 101 *Hygiene 101*
2 cards (101x

Session 1

FOUNDATIONS—Textbook—a work course—*use books in class.*

Nutrition is one of the most fundamental of modern problems. Tragic arrest of a great world movement for human betterment. Should stimulate us to try all the harder.

Consciousness of malnutrition is the result of *modern science.*

The means of correcting malnutrition given us by modern science.

During the last 30 years we have learned the nutritional meaning of an apple as compared with a potato, a peach with an onion, a pork chop with an egg.

Today we can learn to choose food *intelligently* and to ~~study~~ analyze *our nutritional problems.*

The substitution of the word "analyze" for "study" illustrates Mary Swartz Rose's careful choice of words to express fine points of difference and her constant efforts to improve her teaching.

Let us have optimum diets! They are cheaper than sickness, and their effects are from generation to generation—MSR

chapter ten ROSE AT HOME

Mary Swartz Rose kept her home and professional lives from intruding on each other and fulfilled the duties of both admirably. When the setting was home, family and friends she was not self-conscious at being called "Doctor" Rose, but she preferred being called Mrs. Rose by those who knew her; she was a woman, warm and responsive, a friend. As her sister-in-law wrote:

> I have visited in their home often. Mary was a homemaker. Not only did she make her family comfortable and create a family life, but her house was stamped with her personality. She was always improving, adding touches here and there to make it more convenient or more attractive. . . .
>
> She did plan a great deal for him and for the rest of us, especially for the weekends, but we liked her plans. On two or three occasions Anton surprised me by saying a decided "No" to some unimportant suggestions. Mary laughed and agreed with him. As far as I could see, his and Mary's interests were so alike he really had no reason for not agreeing to her plans, but he simply had to prove to himself and to us ever so often that he was his own master. He convinced me he was![1]

The Rose home "Roserock" was on the slope of the Palisades at Edgewater on the west bank of the Hudson River, and was set in a beautiful garden.

The garden was terraced with attractive stone walls, covered with

REFERENCES

CHAPTER 1

1 Interview with Mr. and Mrs. Richard C. Rose, August 3, 1977, Rutland, Vermont.

2 Ben Douglas, *History of the Lawyers of Wayne County, Ohio, from 1812–1900* (Wooster, Ohio, 1900).

3 Interview with Mr. and Mrs. Richard C. Rose, August 3, 1977, Rutland, Vermont.

4 Personal papers of Mr. Richard C. Rose. Letters of recommendation of Miss Mary Davies Swartz.

5 Grace MacLeod, "Mary Swartz Rose," *Journal of Home Economics* 33: 221, 1941.

6 Henry C. Sherman, "Mary Swartz Rose—An Appreciation," *Journal of Nutrition* 21: 209, 1941.

7 Harold H. Williams, "The Founding of the American Institute of Nutrition, Including Commentaries on the Founders," *Federation Proceedings* 36: 1915, 1977.

8 Mary de Garmo Bryan, "Some Dimensions in Food and Nutrition in a Half-Century Since Mary Swartz Rose Came to Teachers College." Lecture before the Greater New York Dietetic Association, April 24, 1964.

9 Remarks by Dr. Henry C. Sherman, October 31, 1939.

10 "A Democratic Scientist," *Forecast,* March 1941.

11 E. Neige Todhunter, "Some Classics of Nutrition and Dietetics," *Journal of American Dietetic Association* 44: 100, 1964.

12 "Presentation of First Mary Swartz Rose Fellowship (by Clara Mae Taylor) to Pearl Jackson," *Journal of American Dietetic Association* 25: 1029, 1949.

13 Clara Mae Taylor, "Reminiscences of Mary Swartz Rose." Conference on Education in Nutrition—Looking Forward from the Past, February 26 and 27, 1974, at Teachers College, Columbia University.

14 Sherman, "Mary Swartz Rose 1874–1941," *Journal of Biological Chemistry* 140: 687, 1941.

15 Remarks by Dr. Grace MacLeod at presentation of portrait, 1936.
16 MacLeod, "Mary Swartz Rose."

CHAPTER 2

1 Clara May Taylor, "Reminiscences of Mary Swartz Rose." Conference on Education in Nutrition—Looking Forward from the Past, February 26 and 27, 1974, at Teachers College, Columbia University.
2 ———, "A Picture of Mary Swartz Rose." Comments at Academy of Medicine, New York, 1950.
3 Ibid.
4 Interview with Dr. Bertlyn Bosley, November 15, 1977, Washington, D.C.
5 Interview with Dr. Esther Phipard, November 7, 1977, MacLean, Va.
6 Personal correspondence of Mrs. Gertrude Gates Mudge, August 30, 1977.
7 Personal correspondence of Mary Swartz Rose to her husband, November 8, 1918.
8 Personal correspondence of Laura T. Rose, sister-in-law of Mary Swartz Rose, February 8, 1942.
9 Ibid.
10 Personal correspondence of Dr. Emma S. Weigley, October 20, 1977.
11 Personal correspondence of Laura T. Rose.
12 Clyde B. Schuman, "Mary Swartz Rose, Scientist and Educator" (Doctoral thesis, New York University, 1945).
13 Personal correspondence of Laura T. Rose.
14 Interview with Dr. and Mrs. Hans W. Vahlteich (Ella McCollum Vahlteich), November 16, 1977, Fort Lee, New Jersey.

CHAPTER 3

1 J. H. Breasted, "The Rise of Man," *Science* 74: 639, 1931.
2 Graham Lusk, "Clio Medica," vol. 10, *Nutrition* (New York: Hoeber, 1933).
3 Clara Mae Taylor and Orrea Florence Pye, *Foundations of Nutrition*, 6 ed. (New York: Macmillan, 1966).
4 Lusk, "Clio Medica."
5 Taylor and Pye, *Foundations of Nutrition*.
6 Lusk, "Clio Medica."
7 Taylor and Pye, *Foundations of Nutrition*.

8 Karl Thomas, "Justus von Liebig, an editorial review," *Journal of Nutrition* 7: 3, 1934.

9 E. Neige Todhunter, "Nutrition Education: Its History, Progress and Problems." Presented as the Mary Swartz Rose Memorial Lecture, April 22, 1965, New York.

10 Lusk, "Clio Medica."

11 Taylor and Pye, *Foundations of Nutrition.*

12 Elmer V. McCollum, *A History of Nutrition* (Boston: Houghton Mifflin, 1957).

13 Russell H. Chittenden, *Development of Physiological Chemistry in the United States,* The Chemical Catalog Company, 1930.

14 Donald B. Tower, "Neurochemistry—One Hundred Years, 1875–1975," *Annals of Neurology* 1: 2, 1977.

15 Elmer V. McCollum, "Biographical Memoir of Stanley Rossiter Benedict," *Biographical Memoirs* 27, 7th memoir (Washington, D.C.: National Academy of Science, 1952).

16 Williamina S. Himwich, "Lafayette B. Mendel and His Scientific Ancestry," in *Essays on History of Nutrition and Dietetics,* comp. Adelia M. Beeuwkes, E. Neige Todhunter, and Emma S. Weigley (Chicago: American Dietetic Association, 1967).

17 McCollum, "My Early Experiences in the Study of Foods and Nutrition," *Annual Review of Biochemistry* 22: 1, 1953.

18 William C. Rose, "Recollections of Personalities Involved in the Early History of American Biochemistry," *Nutrition Reviews* 35: 85, 1977.

19 McCollum, "My Early Experiences in the Study of Foods and Nutrition."

20 Ibid.

21 Interview with Mr. and Mrs. Richard C. Rose, August 3, 1977, Rutland, Vermont.

22 William C. Rose, "The Sequence of Events Leading to the Establishment of the Amino Acid Needs of Man," *American Journal of Public Health* 58: 2020, 1968.

23 McCollum, "Biographical Memoir of Stanley Rossiter Benedict."

24 Mary Davies Swartz, "Nutrition Investigation on the Carbohydrates of Lichens, Algae and Related Substances, *Transactions of the Connecticut Academy of Arts and Sciences* 16: 247, 1911.

25 Lafayette B. Mendel and Mary Davies Swartz, "The Physiological Utilization of Some Complex Carbohydrates," *American Journal of Medical Sciences,* March 1910.

26 Franklin C. Bing, "Dietary Fiber—in Historical Perspective," *Journal of American Dietetic Association* 69: 498, 1976.

27 Ibid.

CHAPTER 4

1 Orrea F. Pye, "The Nutrition Program at Teachers College, Columbia University," Conference on Education in Nutrition—Looking Forward from the Past, February 26 and 27, 1974, at Teachers College, Columbia University.

2 James E. Russell, "The Functions of the University in Training Teachers," *Columbia University Quarterly* 1: 335, 1898–99.

3 Charles Glen King, "Reminiscences of Henry C. Sherman." Conference on Education in Nutrition—Looking Forward from the Past, February 26 and 27, 1974.

4 Ibid.

5 E. Neige Todhunter, "Some Classics of Nutrition and Dietetics," *Journal of the American Dietetic Association* 44: 100, 1964.

6 P. L. Day, "Biography of Henry Clapp Sherman," *Journal of Nutrition* 61: 3, 1957.

7 Harold H. Williams, "The Founding of the American Institute of Nutrition, Including Commentaries on the Founders," *Federation Proceedings* 36: 1915, 1977.

8 Mary Swartz Rose, *A Laboratory Handbook for Dietetics* (New York: Macmillan, 1912).

9 Clyde B. Schuman, "Mary Swartz Rose, Scientist and Educator" (Doctoral thesis, New York University, 1945).

10 Clara Mae Taylor, "Grace MacLeod—A Biographical Sketch," *Journal of Nutrition* 95: 1, 1968.

11 Ibid.

12 Ibid.

13 Taylor, "Reminiscences of Mary Swartz Rose." Conference on Education in Nutrition—Looking Forward from the Past.

14 Rose, "University Teaching of Nutrition and Dietetics in the United States," *Nutrition Abstracts and Reviews* 4: 439, 1935.

15 School of Household Arts, Teachers College, *Annotated List of Books Relating to Household Arts*, Teachers College, Columbia University, 1910.

16 Henry C. Sherman, *Chemistry of Food and Nutrition*, (New York: Macmillan, 1911).

17 ———, *Nutritional Improvement of Life*, (New York: Columbia University Press, 1950).

18 Rose, *A Laboratory Handbook for Dietetics*.

19 ———, *The Foundations of Nutrition* (New York: Macmillan, 1927, 1933, and 1938).

20 *College Book News* (New York: Macmillan, undated).

21 Rose and Clara Mae Taylor, "*Food Values of Recipes in Shares and Vitamin Units,*" (New York: Bureau of Publications, Teachers College, Columbia University, 1931 and 1936).
22 Clara Mae Taylor, *Food Values in Shares and Weights* (New York: Macmillan, 1942 and 1959).

CHAPTER 5

1 Henry C. Sherman, Remarks at Presentation of the Associated Grocery Manufacturers of America Award to Mary Swartz Rose, New York, October 31, 1939.
2 Mary Swartz Rose, "University Teaching of Nutrition and Dietetics in the United States," *Nutrition Abstracts and Reviews* 4: 439, 1935.
3 Clara Mae Taylor, "A Tribute to Our Teacher, Mary Swartz Rose." Radio Station WGR, New York, March 27, 1941.
4 Clyde B. Schuman, "Mary Swartz Rose, Scientist and Educator" (Doctoral thesis, New York University, 1945).
5 Elmer V. McCollum, "My Early Experiences in the Study of Foods and Nutrition," *Annual Review of Biochemistry* 22: 1, 1953.
6 ———, "The Beginnings of Essential Nutrition," *Nutrition Reviews,* 14: 257, 1956.
7 Schuman, "Mary Swartz Rose, Scientist and Educator."
8 Lafayette B. Mendel and Mary Davies Swartz, "The Physiological Utilization of Some Complex Carbohydrates," *American Journal of Medical Sciences,* March 1910.
9 Rose, "Some Applications to Our Newer Knowledge of Nutrition," *Teachers College Record* 23, no. 1, 1922, pp. 34–50.
10 Sherman, *Chemistry of Food and Nutrition* (New York: Macmillan, 1911).
11 T. B. Osborne and L. B. Mendel, "The Relation of Growth to the Chemical Constituents of the Diet," *Journal of Biological Chemistry* 15: 311, 1913.
12 ———, "The Inorganic Elements in Nutrition," *Journal of Biological Chemistry* 34: 131, 1918.
13 Sherman in cooperation with Anton R. Rose et al., "Phosphorus Requirement of Maintenance in Man," *Journal of Biological Chemistry* 41: 173, 1920.
14 Sherman in cooperation with Anton R. Rose and Mary Swartz Rose, "Calcium Requirement of Maintenance in Man," *Journal of Biological Chemistry* 44: 21, 1920.
15 Rose, Rena S. Eckman, Edith D. Brownell, Edith Hawley, and Ella Woods, "Experiments on the Utilization of the Calcium of Carrots by Man," *Journal of Biological Chemistry* 41: 349, 1920.

16 ——— and Grace MacLeod, "Experiments on the Utilization of the Calcium of Almonds by Man," *Journal of Biological Chemistry* 57: 305, 1923.
17 Schuman, "Mary Swartz Rose, Scientist and Educator."
18 Rose and Ella McCollum Vahlteich, "Factors in Food Influencing Hemoglobin Regeneration, I. Whole Wheat Flour, White Flour, Prepared Bran and Oatmeal," *Journal of Biological Chemistry* 96: 593, 1932.
19 ——— and Lan-Chen Kung, "Factors in Food Influencing Hemoglobin Regeneration, II. Liver in Comparison with Whole Wheat and Prepared Bran," *Journal of Biological Chemistry* 98: 417, 1932.
20 Rose, Vahlteich, and MacLeod, "Factors in Food Influencing Hemoglobin Regeneration, III. Eggs in Comparison with Whole Wheat, Prepared Bran, Oatmeal, Beef Liver and Beef Muscle," *Journal of Biological Chemistry* 104: 217, 1934.
21 ——— and Helen Jackson Hubbell, "The Influence of Sex on Iron Utilization in Rats," *Journal of Nutrition* 15: 91, 1938.
22 Vahlteich, Esther H. Funnell, MacLeod, and Rose, "Egg Yolk and Bran as Sources of Iron in the Human Dietary," *Journal of American Dietetic Association* 11: 331, 1935.
23 Rose, "Iron in the Diet of Normal Children," *American Journal of Public Health* 17: 89, 1927.
24 ———, Vahlteich, Robb, and Emily M. Bloomfield, "Iron Requirement in Early Childhood," *Journal of Nutrition* 3: 229, 1930.
25 Rose and McCollum, "Studies in Nutrition, II. The Effect of Adding Egg to a Diet Already Adequate," *Journal of Biological Chemistry* 78: 549, 1928.
26 Franklin C. Bing, "Assaying the Availability of Iron," *Journal of American Dietetic Association* 60: 114, 1972.
27 Rose and Esther Funnell Phipard, "Vitamin B and G Values of Peas and Lima Beans under Various Conditions," *Journal of Nutrition* 14: 55, 1937.
28 Robb, Vahlteich, and Rose, "Vitamin B_1 Intake of Nursery School Children," *American Journal of Diseases of Children* 55: 544, 1938.
29 Schuman, "Mary Swartz Rose, Scientist and Educator."
30 Ibid.
31 Ibid.
32 Ibid.
33 Rose and Harriet C. Jacobson, "A Dietary Study in a Children's Hospital," *Teachers College Bulletin* 13, February 1912.
34 ———, Cora E. Gray, and Katherine Foster, "The Relation of Diet to Health and Growth of Children in Institutions," *Child Development Monograph 2, 1930.*
35 ———, Robb, and Gertrude M. Borgeson, "The Food Consumption of Nursery School Children," *Child Development* 3: 29, 1932.

36 ——— and Emma W. Gardner, "The Banana as a Food for the Aged," *Journal of American Dietetic Association* 16: 208, 1940.

CHAPTER 6

1 Mary Swartz Rose, "Nutrition and the Health of the School Child," *Journal of American Dietetic Association* 15: 63, 1939.
2 ———, "The Training of the School Dietitian," *The Psychologic Clinic* 6: 52, 1912.
3 E. Neige Todhunter, "Nutrition Education: Its History, Progress and Problems." Presented as the Mary Swartz Rose Memorial Lecture, April 22, 1965, New York.
4 Ellen H. Richards, *First Lessons in Food and Diet* (Boston: Whitcomb and Barrows, 1904).
5 ———, *Good Luncheons for Rural Schools without Kitchens* (Boston: Whitcomb and Barrows, 1906).
6 Rose, "The Feeding of Young Children," *Teachers College Bulletin,* 2nd series, no. 10, 1911.
7 ———, "Lessons on Food and Nutrition." School of Practical Arts Emergency Courses, Teachers College, Columbia University, May 1917.
8 ———, "The Health Program at P. S. 43."
9 ——— and Gertrude Gates Mudge, "A Nutrition Class, in Cooperation with a Summer Play School," *Journal of Home Economics* 12: 49, 1920.
10 Charles H. Smith, *How to Conduct a Nutrition Class* (New York: Child Health Organization, 1918).
11 Rose, "Recent Developments in Child Feeding," *Teachers College Record* 21: 470, 1920.
12 ———, *Teaching Nutrition to Boys and Girls* (New York: Macmillan, 1932).
13 ———, "Food Lessons for Nutrition Classes," *Teachers College Bulletin* 41, May 1922.
14 Jeanette Garrett, "The Story of the 'Getsick' and 'Keepwell' Families" (nutrition lessons directed by Mary Swartz Rose and Cora M. Winchell) *American Food Journal,* May 1925.
15 Julia K. Cowles, with a foreword by Mary Swartz Rose, "Food Families in Food Town. Teaching Nutrition to Fourth Grade Children," *American Food Journal,* April 1925.
16 Rose, "A Five-Year Study of Nutrition Teaching in the Fifth and Sixth Grades of the Elementary School," *Teachers College Record* 31: 733, 1930.
17 Personal papers of Mary Swartz Rose, "Lessons in Food and Nutrition."
18 Ibid.
19 Ibid.

20 Rose and Bertlyn Bosley, "Vegetables to Help Us Grow—A Nutrition Unit for the First, Second, and Third Grades of the Elementary School" (New York: Bureau of Publications, Teachers College, Columbia University, 1941).
21 ———, "Feeding Our Teeth—A Nutrition Unit for the Third and Fourth Grades of the Elementary School" (New York: Bureau of Publications, Teachers College, Columbia University, 1940).
22 ———, "Our Cereals—A Nutrition Unit for the Fourth, Fifth, and Sixth Grades of the Elementary School" (New York: Bureau of Publications, Teachers College, Columbia University, 1938).
23 Todhunter, "Nutrition Education: Its History, Progress and Problems."
24 Rose, "Nutrition and the Health of the School Child," *Journal of American Dietetic Association* 15: 63, 1939.
25 Rose, "Has Nutrition Found Its Rightful Place in Education?" *New York State Education*, June 1926.
26 ———, *Teaching Nutrition to Boys and Girls.*
27 ——— and Bertlyn Bosley, "A Nutrition Program for the Elementary Grades," *Forecast* 55: 322, 1939.
28 ———, "University Teaching of Nutrition and Dietetics in the United States," *Nutrition Abstracts and Reviews* 4: 439, 1935.
29 ———, "Our Children and Their Nutrition Needs," *Teachers College Record* 33: 391, 1932.

CHAPTER 7

1 E. Neige Todhunter, "Some Classics of Nutrition and Dietetics," *Journal of American Dietetic Association* 44: 100, 1964.
2 Personal correspondence of Mary Swartz Rose to her husband, November 12 and December 5, 1918.
3 Clyde B. Schuman, "Mary Swartz Rose, Scientist and Educator" (Doctoral thesis, New York University, 1945).
4 Life Extension Institute, *Food, Fuel for the Human Engine,* New York, 1917.
5 Mary Swartz Rose, Mary G. McCormick, and Marion F. Walker, "Living on Twenty-five Cents a Day," *Teachers College Record* 19: 269, 1918.
6 Bibliography Committee, New York Nutrition Council, *Nutrition Bibliography* (New York: Health Division, American Red Cross, 1921 and 1923).
7 Committee on Economic Standards, New York Nutrition Council, *Good Nutrition and Adequate Food Allowances for the Family* (New York: Nutrition Council, 1922).
8 Personal papers of Mary Swartz Rose. Newspaper articles.
9 Rose, "How Much Meat?" *Good Housekeeping,* January 1910.
10 ———, "Some Food Facts to Help the Housewife in Feeding the Fam-

ily," *Technical Education Bulletin* 27, Teachers College, Columbia University, New York, 1916.
11 ———, *The Children's Food* (New York: The Emergency Committee of the American Home Economics Association, New York Section, 1917).
12 ——— with Mary G. McCormick and Irma A. Latzer, "How to Plan Meals in War Time with Economical Menus and Suggestions for Marketing," *Technical Education Bulletin* 33, Teachers College, Columbia University, New York, 1917.
13 ———, *Everyday Foods in War Time* (New York: Macmillan, 1918).
14 ———, "Some Applications of our Newer Knowledge of Nutrition," *Teachers College Record* 23: 34, 1922.
15 ———, "Racial Food Habits in Relation to Health," *The Scientific Monthly* 44: 257, 1937.
16 ———, *Feeding the Family* (New York: Macmillan, 1st ed., 1916).
17 ———, 3rd ed., 1929 and 4th ed., 1940.
18 Personal correspondence of Mary Swartz Rose, April 8, 1940.
19 ———, December 15, 1939.
20 Interview with Miss Helen Stacey, July 27, 1977, Washington, D.C.

CHAPTER 8

1 Mary Swartz Rose, "Nutrition as an International Problem."
2 *Report of the Technical Commission on Nutrition on the Work of Its Third Session, 1939.* Bulletin of the Health Organization of the League of Nations, vol. 7, extract no. 8.
3 Personal papers of Mr. Richard C. Rose. Unpublished address of Mary Swartz Rose, "Nutrition Activities of the League of Nations," 1936.
4 Clara Mae Taylor, "A Picture of Mary Swartz Rose." Comments at Academy of Medicine, New York, 1950.
5 Personal correspondence of Mary Swartz Rose, July 6, 1939.
6 Letter from Mary Swartz Rose to Dr. Hazel K. Stiebeling, October 19, 1937.
7 Mary Swartz Rose, "The Effect of Quick Freezing on the Nutritive Values of Foods," *Journal of the American Medical Association* 114: 1356, 1940.
8 Report of Council on Foods and Nutrition, *Journal of the American Medical Association* 116: 2401, 1941.
9 Clyde B. Schuman, "Mary Swartz Rose, Scientist and Educator" (Doctoral thesis, New York University, 1945).
10 Henry C. Sherman, Remarks at Presentation of the Associated Grocery Manufacturers of America Award to Mary Swartz Rose, New York, October 31, 1939.
11 Ibid.

12 Schuman, "Mary Swartz Rose, Scientist and Educator."
13 "Presentation of First Mary Swartz Rose Fellowship (by Clara Mae Taylor) to Pearl Jackson," *Journal of American Dietetic Association* 25: 1029, 1949.
14 Schuman, "Mary Swartz Rose, Scientist and Educator."
15 Personal papers of Mr. Richard C. Rose. Unpublished address of Mary Swartz Rose, "World Movements in Nutrition," 1940.
16 Rose, "Recent Developments in Child Feeding," *Teachers College Record* 21: 470, 1920.
17 ———, "Nutrition in the Life of the Growing Child," *Journal of Home Economics* 26: 533, 1934.
18 ———, "Child Nutrition and Diet," *Journal of Home Economics* 15: 129, 1923.
19 ———, "Recent Developments in Child Feeding."
20 ———, "The Question of Child Feeding," *The Modern Hospital* 13, no. 5, 1919.
21 ———, "What Is Progress in Nutrition?" *Journal of Home Economics* 17: 372, 1925.
22 ———, "Child Nutrition and Diet."

CHAPTER 9

1 Nicholas Murray Butler, "Annual Report of the President, 1908–09." Columbia University, New York.
2 "The Aims and Activities of the Department of Nutrition," *Teachers College Record* 16: 90, 1915.
3 Clara Mae Taylor, "Reminiscences of Mary Swartz Rose." Conference on Education in Nutrition—Looking Forward from the Past, February 26 and 27, 1974, at Teachers College, Columbia University.
4 Clyde B. Schuman, "Mary Swartz Rose, Scientist and Educator" (Doctoral thesis, New York University, 1945).
5 Ibid.
6 Grace Macleod, "Mary Swartz Rose, Pioneer in Nutrition," *American Cookery* 49: 37, 1944.
7 Henry C. Sherman, "Mary Swartz Rose—An Appreciation," *Journal of Nutrition* 21: 209, 1941.
8 Schuman, "Mary Swartz Rose, Scientist and Educator."
9 Personal correspondence of Dr. Hazel K. Stiebeling, September 6, 1977.
10 Personal correspondence of Dr. Natalie K. Fitch, September, 3, 1977.
11 Personal correspondence of Mrs. Katherine Wisely, August 20, 1977.
12 Personal correspondence of Mrs. Pauline Murrah Benz, December 13, 1977.

13 Personal correspondence of Dr. Doris S. Runciman, March 5, 1978.
14 Maurice A. Bigelow, director of the School of Practical Arts, as cited in Schuman, "Mary Swartz Rose, Scientist and Educator"

CHAPTER 10

1 Personal correspondence of Laura T. Rose, sister-in-law of Mary Swartz Rose, February 8, 1942.
2 *The New York Sun,* May 12, 1918.
3 Personal correspondence of Dr. and Mrs. Hans W. Vahlteich (Ella McCollum Vahlteich), March 3, 1978.

EPILOGUE

1 L. A. Cremin, D. A. Shannon, and M. E. Townsend, *A History of Teachers College, Columbia University* (New York: Columbia University Press, 1954), pp. 56–57.
2 Bertlyn Bosley and Grace MacLeod, "Establishing Good Food Habits in Gifted Children—A Report of a Study Conducted at Speyer School," *Teachers College Record* 43: 57–70, 1941.

PUBLICATIONS OF MARY SWARTZ ROSE

1910

"The Physiological Utilization of Some Complex Carbohydrates" (as Swartz, with Lafayette B. Mendel, senior author), *American Journal of Medical Sciences* 49: 422–26.

*"How Much Meat?" (as Swartz), *Good Housekeeping 50: 106–9.*

1911

"Nutrition Investigation on the Carbohydrates of Lichens, Algae, and Related Substances" (as Swartz), *Transactions of Connecticut Academy of Arts and Sciences* 16: 247–382.

†"The Feeding of Young Children," *Teachers College Bulletin,* 2nd series no. 10, 10 pp.

"Some Problems in Dietetics," *Household Arts Review* 3: 7–13.

1912

†*A Laboratory Handbook for Dietetics* (New York, Macmillan), pp. viii and 127.

†"A Dietary Study in a Children's Hospital" (with Harriet Jacobson), *Teachers College Bulletin,* 3rd series, no. 13, 16 pp.

"Nutritive Value of Seaweeds," *Journal of Home Economics* 4: 140–45.

"What Anaesthesia Has Done for Surgery," *Woman's Medical Journal* 22: 106–8.

*"How a Knowledge of Food Values Will Help the Housewife to Reduce the Cost of Living," New York State Department of Agriculture *Bulletin* no. 35, 1187–93.

**Popular or semipopular*

†*Cited as books by the Library of Congress, Washington, D.C.*

Bibliographies of Home Economics Literature, nos. 1, 2, and 3, *Journal of Home Economics* 4: 84–89, 174–78, and 297–300.

Bibliographies of Current Home Economics Literature, nos. 4 and 5, *Journal of Home Economics* 4: 369, 371, and 499–502.

"The Training of the School Dietitian," *The Psychologic Clinic* 6: 52–55.

1914

†"Food for School Boys and Girls," *Teachers College Bulletin*, 5th series, no. 12, 15 pp.

1916

†*Feeding the Family* (New York, Macmillan), pp. xv and 449.

†"Some Food Facts to Help the Housewife in Feeding the Family," *Teachers College Bulletin*, 7th series, no. 17, 6 pp.

1917

†"Economical Diet and Cookery in Time of Emergency" (with Cora Winchell and Bertha Shapely), *Teachers College Bulletin*, 8th series, nos. 17 and 18, 15 pp.

†"How to Plan Meals in War Time" (with Mary McCormick and Irma Latzer) *Teachers College Technical Education Bulletin* no. 33, 15 pp.

†The Children's Food (with Geraldine Gorton) (New York; American Home Economics Association Emergency Committee), 10 pp.

"Redundant Sigmoid," *Woman's Medical Journal*, 27: 112.

"The Biological Efficiency of Potato Nitrogen" (with Lenna Cooper), *Journal of Biological Chemistry*, 30: 201–4.

"Creatinuria in Women," *Journal of Biological Chemistry* 32: 1–6.

*"Wheat Substitutes" (with Robert Chaddock, Henry C. Sherman, and May Van Arsdale), *Columbia War Papers*, series 1, no. 15, pp. 1-22.

*"The Same Nourishment for Less Money," *Ladies' Home Journal* 34: 70–71.

1918

†*Everyday Foods in War Time* (reprinted in part from the *Farmer's Wife*) (New York, Macmillan), pp. viii and 117.

*"My Husband Won't Eat It," *Ladies' Home Journal*, 35: 33.

*"Living on Twenty-five Cents a Day" (with Mary McCormick and Marion Walker), *Teachers College Record* 19: 269–77.

*"Team Work in Food Conservation," *American Woman's Magazine* 1: 134–36.

1919

"On the Utilization of Salep Mannan," *Proceedings of Society for Experimental Biology and Medicine* 17: 7–9.

"The Utilization of the Calcium of Carrots by Man," *Proceedings of Society for Experimental Biology and Medicine* 17: 66.

"The Question of Child Feeding," *The Modern Hospital* 13: 435–40.

1920

†"Recent Developments in Child Feeding," *Teachers College Bulletin,* 12th series, no. 4, 16 pp.

"Experiments on the Utilization of the Calcium of Carrots by Man" (with the cooperation of R. Eckman, E. Brownell, E. Hawley, and E. Woods), *Journal of Biological Chemistry* 41: 349–55.

"Experiments on the Utilization of Salep Mannan" (with Louise Browne, Lucy Gillett, E. Rothermel and H. Coombs), *Journal of Biological Chemistry* 42: 159–66.

"Calcium Requirement of Maintenance in Man" (with Henry C. Sherman, senior author, and Anton R. Rose), *Journal of Biological Chemistry* 34: 21–27.

"Some Human Digestion Experiments with Raw White of Egg" (with Grace MacLeod), *Proceedings of Society for Experimental Biology and Medicine* 17: 199–20 and *Journal of Biological Chemistry* 50: 83–88, 1922.

"A Nutrition Class in Co-operation with a Summer Play School" (with Gertrude Gates Mudge), *Journal of Home Economics* 12: 49–58.

"Recent Developments in Child Feeding," *Teachers College Record* 21: 470–84.

1921

†*A Laboratory Handbook for Dietetics,* 2nd ed. (New York: Macmillan), pp. xii and 158.

†"The Child's Day, An Entertainment to Impress Daily Habits for Healthy Life" (with Geraldine Gorton), *Teachers College Bulletin,* 13th series, no. 2, 16 pp.

†"Some Food Facts to Help the Housewife in Feeding the Family," 2nd ed., *Teachers College Bulletin*, 12th series, no. 11, 7 pp.

1922

†"Food Lessons for Nutrition Classes," *Teachers College Bulletin,* 13th series, no. 11, 26 pp.

"Diet in Tuberculosis," *The Commonwealth,* Massachusetts, vol. 9, no. 4.

"Some Experiments on the Digestibility of Rolled Oats Prepared in Various Ways," *Journal of Home Economics* 14: 9–14.

"Food and Food Values," *Woman's Medical Journal* 29: 70–76.

"The Almond as a Source of the A Vitamin" (with Grace MacLeod), *Proceedings of Society for Experimental Biology and Medicine* 19: 391–93.

"The Basal Metabolism of Girls from Eleven to Fourteen Years of Age" (with Grace MacLeod), *Proceedings,* American Physiological Society, Toronto, Canada and *The American Journal of Physiology* 63: 399–400, 1923.

"Some Applications of Our Newer Knowledge of Nutrition," *Teachers College Record* 23: 34–51.

1923

"Experiments on the Utilization of the Calcium of Almonds by Man" (with Grace MacLeod), *Journal of Biological Chemistry* 57: 305–15.

"Digestion Experiments with the Raw White of Egg. II. The Digestibility of Unbeaten in Comparison with Beaten White" (with Grace MacLeod), *Journal of Biological Chemistry* 63: 369–71.

"Maintenance Values for the Proteins of Milk, Bread and Milk, Meat, and Soy Bean Curd in Human Nutrition" (with Grace MacLeod and B. Bisbey), *Proceedings of Society for Experimental Biology and Medicine* 21: 143–44.

"Child Nutrition and Diet," *Journal of Home Economics* 15: 129–42.

"How to Meet the Problem of the Delicate Child," *Nation's Health* 5: 777–78, 843.

*"Wise Buying of Food," *Modern Priscilla,* 23: 22, 36, and 41.

1924

†*Feeding the Family,* 2nd ed. (New York, Macmillan) pp. xix and 487.

"Teaching Nutrition to Third Grade Children" (with Catherine Newton), *The American Food Journal* 19: 414–15.

*"The High Cost of Growing," *Hygeia* 2: 343–46.

1925

†"Nutrition in an Elementary School" (with Helen Knowlton), *Teachers College Bulletin*, 16th series, no. 12, 46 pp.

"Maintenance Values for the Proteins of Milk, Meat, Bread and Milk, and Soy Bean Curd" (with Grace MacLeod), *Journal of Biological Chemistry* 66: 847–67.

"A Comparison of the Basal Metabolism of Normal Women with Present Prediction Standards" (with Grace MacLeod), *The American Journal of Physiology,* 72: 236–37.

"What Is Progress in Nutrition?" *Journal of Home Economics* 17: 372–77 and 442–48.

"Nutrition in an Elementary School," *The American Food Journal* 20: 594–96.
*"Food After Forty," *Hygeia* 3: 363–65.

1926

"The Influence of Prolonged Administration of Egg Upon the Hemoglobin Content of Children's Blood," *Journal of Biological Chemistry* 67: xx–xxi.
"Some Factors Influencing the Basal Metabolism of Children" (with Grace MacLeod), *Journal of Biological Chemistry* 67: xix–xx.
"Ten Years of Vitamin Research," *Journal of Home Economics* 18: 248–53 and 306–16.
"Has Nutrition Found Its Rightful Place in Education?" *New York State Teachers Journal* 13: 651–57.
*"Is the Study of Nutrition Worth While?" *Discobolus* 3: 3–4, 10–12.
*"The Nutrition Classes of the Health Experiment," *P. S. 157 The John Hancock News*, vol. 2, no. 2, 10.

1927

†*Foundations of Nutrition* (New York: Macmillan), pp. xi and 501.
"Iron in the Diet of Normal Children," *American Journal of Public Health* 17: 89–91 and *Experiment Station Record* 57: 688–89.
"What Metabolic Research Has Taught in Nutrition of Children," *Nation's Health* 9: 21–23.
*"A Health Experiment in Miss Goodhart's Room," *P. S. 157 The John Hancock News*, vol. 2, no. 2, 11.
"A Health Experiment in Harlem," *Food and Health Education* 22: 45.
*"What Sweets Shall Children Have?" *Ladies' Home Journal* 44: 171.

1928

†"Choosing Food for Health," *Handbook on Positive Health* (editor, Lenna Meanes), rev. ed., chap. IV (New York: Women's Foundation for Health), pp. 110–32.
"Supplementary Values Among Foods. I. Adding Egg to an Adequate Diet Compared with Increasing Vegetables" (with Ella McCollum), *Proceedings of Society for Experimental Biology and Medicine* 25: 697–98.
"Studies in Nutrition. I. Growth, Reproduction, and Lactation on Diets with Different Proportions of Cereals and Vegetables" (with Ella McCollum Vahlteich and Grace MacLeod), *Journal of Biological Chemistry* 78: 535–47.
"Studies in Nutrition. II. The Effect of Adding Egg to a Diet Already Adequate" (with Ella McCollum Vahlteich, R. E. Evans, and Emily Bloomfield), *Journal of Biological Chemistry* 78: 549–55 and *United States Egg and Poultry Magazine* 16: 51–54, 1930.

"Supplementary Values Among Foods. II. Growth and Reproduction on White Bread with Various Supplements" (with Grace MacLeod), *The Journal of Nutrition* 1: 29–38.

"Visualizing Food Values" (with Margaret Hessler, Hazel Stiebeling, and Clara Mae Taylor), *Journal of Home Economics* 20: 781–87.

*"What Are Green Vegetables?" *Ladies' Home Journal* 45: 52 and 56.

*"Foods That Go Together," *Ladies' Home Journal* 45: 89–90.

*"The Baby's Automobile Kit," *Ladies' Home Journal* 45: 42–44.

*"What About Dried Fruits?" *Ladies' Home Journal* 45: 101.

1929

†*Feeding the Family,* 3rd ed. (New York: Macmillan), pp. xv and 459.

†*A Laboratory Handbook for Dietetics,* 3rd ed. (New York: Macmillan), pp. xiv and 269.

"Influence of Whole Wheat Upon Hemoglobin Regeneration in Albino Rats (with Ella McCollum Vahlteich and Emily Bloomfield)," *Proceedings of Society for Experimental Biology and Medicine* 26: 322–23.

"What Place Have Aluminum, Copper, Manganese and Zinc in Normal Nutrition?" *The Journal of Nutrition* 1: 541–56.

"Nutrition in Health Education" *Oregon Education Journal* 3: 6, 21–22, and 31.

*"Do You Agree with Your Food?" *Ladies' Home Journal* 46: 96 and 113.

*"When My Boy Goes to College, Who Will Feed Him?" *Ladies' Home Journal* 46: 122–24.

1930

†*Foundations of Nutrition,* 2nd ed. (New York, Macmillan), pp. xi and 501.

†"The Relation of Diet to Health and Growth of Children in Institutions, with a Method of Evaluating Dietaries and a Three-Weeks Dietary Conforming to the Standards Proposed" (with Cora Gray and the cooperation of Katherine Foster), Child Development Monograph 2 (New York: Teachers College, Columbia University), pp. vii and 128.

"Functions of Vitamins in Normal Nutrition," *International Clinics* 3: 267–77.

"Iron Requirement in Early Childhood" (with Ella McCollum Vahlteich, Elda Robb, and Emily Bloomfield), *The Journal of Nutrition* 3: 229–35.

"A Five-Year Study of Nutrition Teaching in the Fifth and Sixth Grades of the Elementary School," *Teachers College Record* 31: 733–54.

"Old and New Emphases in the Teaching of Nutrition," *Journal of Home Economics* 22: 878–84 and 977–82.

1931

†"Food Values of Recipes in Shares and Vitamin Units" (with Clara Mae Taylor) (New York: Teachers College, Columbia University), 38 pp.

1932

†*Teaching Nutrition to Boys and Girls* (New York: Macmillan), pp. xxiv and 198.

"The Food Consumption of Nursery School Children" (with Elda Robb and Gertrude Borgeson), *Child Development* 3: 29–42.

"The Nutritional Significance of Some Mineral Elements Occurring as Traces in the Animal Body," *The Yale Journal of Biology and Medicine* 4: 499–518.

"Wheat Bran as a Source of Vitamin B" (with Ella McCollum Vahlteich, Esther Funnell, and Grace MacLeod), *Journal of the American Dietetic Association* 7: 369–74.

"Factors in Food Influencing Hemoglobin Regeneration. I. Whole Wheat Flour, White Flour, Prepared Bran, and Oatmeal" (with Ella McCollum Vahlteich), *Journal of Biological Chemistry* 96: 593–608.

"Factors in Food Influencing Hemoglobin Regeneration. II. Liver in Comparison with Whole Wheat and Prepared Bran (with Lan-Chen Kung), *Journal of Biological Chemistry* 98: 417–37.

"The Influence of Bran on the Alimentary Tract" (with Grace MacLeod, Ella McCollum Vahlteich, Esther Funnell, and Catherine Newton), *Journal of the American Dietetic Association* 8: 133–56.

"Our Children and Their Nutrition Needs," *Teachers College Record* 32: 391–401.

1933

"Belief in Magic," *Journal of the American Dietetic Association* 8: 489–503.

1934

"Factors in Food Influencing Hemoglobin Regeneration. III. Eggs in Comparison with Whole Wheat, Prepared Bran, Oatmeal, Beef Liver, and Beef Muscle" (with Ella McCollum Vahlteich and Grace MacLeod), *Journal of Biological Chemistry* 104: 217–29.

"Nutrition in the Life of the Growing Child," *Journal of Home Economics* 16: 533–40.

"Teaching Nutrition to Boys and Girls," *Journal of the National Education Association* 23: 129–31.

1935

†"Child Nutrition on a Low-Priced Diet: With Special Reference to the Supplementary Value of an Egg a Day, the Effect of Adding Orange Juice, and of Replacing Egg by Liver" (with Gertrude M. Borgeson), Child De-

velopment Monographs, no. 17 (New York: Teachers College, Columbia University), pp. xiv and 109.

"Egg Yolk and Bran as Sources of Iron in the Human Dietary" (with Ella McCollum Vahlteich, Esther Funnell, and Grace MacLeod), *Journal of the American Dietetic Association* 11: 331–34.

"University Teaching of Nutrition and Dietetics in the United States," *Nutrition Abstracts and Reviews* 4: 439–45.

1936

†*Food Values of Recipes in Shares and Vitamin Units* 2nd ed. (with Clara Mae Taylor) (New York: Teachers College, Columbia University), 38 pp.

"Effect of Digestibility upon the Availability of Iron in Whole Wheat (with Ella McCollum Vahlteich and Grace MacLeod), *The Journal of Nutrition* 11: 31–36.

"Protein Utilization as Affected by the Presence of Small Amounts of Bran or Its Fiber" (with Esther Funnell, Ella McCollum Vahlteich, Sadie Morris, and Grace MacLeod) *The Journal of Nutrition* 11: 37–45.

"Nutrition as an International Problem," *Journal of the American Dietetic Association* 12: 464.

1937

†*A Laboratory Handbook for Dietetics,* 4th ed. (New York: Macmillan), pp. xi and 322.

"Vitamin B and G Values of Peas and Lima Beans Under Various Conditions" (with Esther Funnell Phipard) *The Journal of Nutrition* 14: 55–67.

"Racial Food Habits in Relation to Health," *The Scientific Monthly* 44: 257–67.

1938

†"Our Cereals. A Nutrition Unit for the Fourth, Fifth, and Sixth Grades of the Elementary School" (with Bertlyn Bosley) (New York: Teachers College, Columbia University), pp. vi and 34.

†*The Foundations of Nutrition,* 3rd ed. (New York: Macmillan), pp. xii and 625.

*"Good Teaching Important If Children Are to Benefit from Knowledge of Nutrition," *Nutrition News* (National Dairy Council), vol. 1, no. 4, 12.

"The Influence of Sex on Iron Utilization in Rats (with Helen Jackson Hubbell)," *The Journal of Nutrition* 15: 91–102.

"Vitamin B_1 Intake of Nursery School Children" (with Ella McCollum Vahlteich and Elda Robb), *American Journal of Diseases of Children* 55: 544–53.

"A Review of Investigations on the Nutritive Value of Eggs" (with Ella McCollum Vahlteich) *Journal of the American Dietetic Association* 14: 593–614.

1939

"Nutrition and the Health of the School Child," *Journal of the American Dietetic Association* 15: 63–85.

"A Nutrition Program for the Elementary Grades" (with Bertlyn Bosley), *Forecast* 55: 322–23, 348, 359, and 367.

"Diet," in *Fit to Teach* (with Clara Mae Taylor), Ninth Yearbook, Department of Classroom Teachers, National Education Association.

1940

†*Feeding the Family,* 4th ed. (New York: Macmillan), pp. xv and 421.

†Feeding Our Teeth. A Nutrition Unit for the Third and Fourth Grades of the Elementary School (with Bertlyn Bosley) (New York: Teachers College, Columbia University), pp. iv and 26.

"The Banana as a Food for the Aged" (with Emma Gardner) *Journal of the American Dietetic Association* 16: 208–14.

"The Effect of Quick-Freezing on the Nutritive Value of Foods," *Journal of the American Medical Association* 114: 1356–61.

*"Protective Foods," in *Neighborhood Health,* New York City, Department of Health, vol. 6, no. 1.

*"Nutrition of Man," *Encyclopedia Americana* 20: 520B

1941

†Vegetables to Help Us Grow. A Nutrition Unit for the First, Second, and Third Grades of the Elementary School (with Bertlyn Bosley) (New York: Teachers College, Columbia University), pp. iv and 25.

BOOK REVIEWS

In *Journal of Home Economics:*
January 1924
page 34 *Girth Control* by H. T. Finck
Right Food the Right Remedy by Charles Froude
The Dietary of Health and Disease by G. I. Thomas
Food for the Diabetic by Mary Pascoe Huddleson
Fasting and Undernutrition by Sergius Morgulis
May 1927
page 281 *Nutrition Work With Children* by Lydia J. Roberts
November 1930
page 925 *Dietetics for High Schools* by Florence Willard and Lucy H. Gillett
In *Progressive Education:*
1927, 4: 335 *Nutrition Work with Children* by Lydia J. Roberts

In *Hospital Social Service:*
1929, 19: 78 *Handbook on Diet* by Eugene E. Marcovici
In *American Journal of Public Health:*
1931
page 458 *Grow Thin on Good Food* by Luella E. Axtell, M.D.

APPENDIX A

ANNOTATED LIST OF BOOKS RELATING TO NUTRITION, 1910

Abderhalden, Emil. *Physiological Chemistry.* Wiley. 722 pp. $5.

A series of lectures not covering all phases of physiological chemistry, but treating in detail and from a very modern point of view, such topics as the different groups of foodstuffs and their nutritive relations, the metabolism of the different organs and of the body as a whole, and some of the more important theories of the relation of physiological chemistry to medicine. It contains a particularly complete account of the modern work on the structure of the proteins.

Armsby, Henry Prentiss. *Principles of Animal Nutrition.* Wiley. 614 pp. $4.

A very complete account, up to about 1903, of what is commonly called the "Statistics of Nutrition," dealing not so much with nutrition processes as with the extent of metabolism under various conditions.

Bunge, G. *Physiological and Pathological Chemistry.* Blakiston. Philadelphia. 470 pp. $3.

A series of lectures presenting some of the most important features of Physiological and Pathological Chemistry in an interesting and vigorous style. The treatment of the subject matter is not always well balanced, and in some respects not up to date, but the suggestiveness of the book makes it valuable to the teacher. Three chapters are of special value: "Milk and the Food of Infants," "The Inorganic Foodstuffs," and "Iron."

Chapin, Henry Dwight, M. D. *Theory and Practice of Infant Feeding.* Wood. 350 pp. $2.25.

A broad treatment of the subject of infant feeding, including considerable discussion of the principles of nutrition, and such related topics as the care of milk and the development of the child. Revised in 1909.

Chittenden, R. H. *Nutrition of Man.* Stokes. 321 pp. $3.

The first part of the book gives a semi-popular account of the nutritive processes; the rest consists of a description and discussion of the author's investigations on the effects of a low protein diet.

Friedenwald & Ruhräh. *Diet in Health and Disease.* Saunders. Philadelphia. 765 pp. $4

The treatment of diet in health is so condensed as to be of little importance, but that of diet in disease is detailed and more authoritative than in any other covering an equal range of diseases.

Friedenwald & Ruhräh. *Dietetics for Nurses.* Saunders. Philadelphia. $1.50.

An abridged and somewhat simplified edition of *Diet in Health and Disease.* This is the best of the small books available as text-books for nurses-in-training.

Gautier, Emile Justin. *Diet and Dietetics.* Lippincott. Philadelphia. 552 pp. $3.50.

An interesting book, which contains a great deal of suggestive material, but the author has not always been careful to select his facts from the most reliable sources, and the translation is sometimes obscure. It gives more attention to the ash constituents than most books on Dietetics.

Gibbs, Winifred S. *Lessons in the Proper Feeding of the Family.* N. Y. Association for Improving the Condition of the Poor, 105 East 22nd Street, N. Y. $ .25.

A small pamphlet by an experienced dietitian, giving very practical suggestions for those of limited time and means. Special attention is given to the proper food for children.

Hammarsten, Olof. *Physiological Chemistry.* Wiley. 1909. 845 pp. $4.

The standard book of reference in physiological chemistry. It is a compendium of statements of the work of various investigators upon still unsettled points, and in reference to original papers, and frequently describes analytical methods. It is a book for intensive study rather than general reading.

Hill, Alexander. *Recent Advances in Physiology and Biochemistry.* Edward Arnold, London.

A collection of monographs by several English physiologists, treating exhaustively such topics as "Enzyme Action," "Purins," and the "Precursors of Urea." The chapters on "Metabolism of Fat," and

"Metabolism of Carbohydrates," and the discussion of total metabolism under heading the "Respiratory Exchange," are particularly valuable to students of nutrition.

Holt, L. Emmett, M. D. *Care and Feeding of Children.* Appleton. 66 pp. $ .75.

A small handbook in the form of a simple catechism, giving practical suggestions for the feeding of children up to the tenth year. The last edition (1909) has been carefully revised and enlarged.

Holt, L. Emmett, M. D. *Diseases of Infancy and Childhood.* Appleton. 1171 pp. $6.

This book is valuable to the student of dietetics for its section on nutrition, in which the subject of infant feeding is treated in great detail; and also for the chapter on "Growth and Development."

Howell, William Henry. *Textbook of Physiology.* Saunders. Philadelphia. 977 pp. $6.

Probably the best of the standard textbooks in physiology for the general student. The discussion of digestion and of the nutritive history of the foodstuffs is interesting and authoritative.

Hull, Winifred S. *Nutrition and Dietetics.* Appleton. $2.50.

A simple and comprehensive treatment of foods and of feeding in both health and disease, the result of the author's experience in teaching classes of nurses. Excellent for this purpose, for a reference book in high school classes, or for study in women's clubs.

Hutchinson, Robert. *Food and Dietetics.* Wood. 1906. 548 pp. $3.

Kerley, Charles Gilmore. *Short Talks to Young Mothers.* Saunders. Philadelphia. 327 pp.

A simple hand-book, in which is embodied much of the information on the general care and nutrition of children found in the "Treatment of Diseases of Children," by the same author.

Kerley, Charles Gilmore. *Treatment of Diseases of Children.* Saunders. Philadelphia. 629 pp. $5.

A thoroughly up-to-date book, noticeable for its endeavor to educate those having the care of children in the importance of prophylactic measures. The chapter on "Nutrition and Growth" presents the subject of artificial feeding in a very clear and simple manner, while giving unusual emphasis on the possibility and desirability of maternal nursing.

Lusk, Graham. *Science of Nutrition.* Saunders. Philadelphia. 402 pp. $2.50.

This book deals with both the statistics of nutrition and the explanation of nutritive processes. It is noticeable for the large amount of experimental data incorporated without making the work a mere compendium. While admirable from a scientific standpoint, it is rather technical for the student of dietetics.

Pattee, Alida F. *Practical Dietetics.* (Author and Publisher, Mt. Vernon, N. Y.). $1.50.

A little book for nurses, containing a simple review of the principles of nutrition, and recipes for practical cookery, for which the fuel values are calculated. It gives plain directions for dietary computations and methods, and includes useful table of the food value of the small quantities used in individual recipes.

Rose, Flora. *Human Nutrition,* Part I and Part II. Cornell Reading Course for Farmers' Wives. Human Nutrition, No. 6. (Free).

Small pamphlet treating the dietary requirements in a very simple way. Part I has a useful table of 100 calorie portions of common food materials. These papers would be valuable for high school classes.

Schaefer, E. A. *Text-book of Physiology.* Macmillan. $8.

The most extended text-bookof Physiology in English, abounding in references to literature. It has not, however, been revised since its original publication in 1898.

Tigerstedt, Robert. *Text-book of Physiology.* Appleton. $4.

A good reference textbook in physiology, especially strong on nutrition and circulation, in both of which subjects the author is high authority.

Von Noorden, Carl. *Metabolism and Practical Medicine.* Keener. Chicago. 452 pp.

The most exhaustive discussion of metabolism which has ever been published. It considers the nutritive requirements and nutritive processes of the body, both in health and disease, with detailed discussion of general disturbances of metabolism in many abnormal conditions. Specific instructions as to feeding are in no case given.

APPENDIX B

As per Clyde B. Schuman's "Mary Swartz Rose, Scientist and Educator," listed below are the students and friends who participated in the Anniversary Dinner for Mary Swartz Rose, held at the time of the New York Meeting of the American Dietetic Association (1936).*

Josephine M. Adams, Lynbrook, N.J.
Mrs. Luise Addis, New York, N.Y.
Esther H. Alden, Philadelphia, Pa.
Lillian Anderson, New York, N.Y.
Grace M. Augustine, Denton, Tex.
Edith M. Barber, New York, N.Y.
Mary I. Barber, Battle Creek, Mich.
Harriet Barto, Urbana, Ill.
Esther L. Batchelder, Kingston, R.I.
Frances Benjamin, New York, N.Y.
Katharine S. Bielby, Salt Lake City, Utah
Jeanette Biggs, Knoxville, Tenn.
Mary Rose Blazek, Montevallo, Ala.
Leila E. Booher, Washington, D.C.
Bertlyn Bosley, New York, N.Y.
Anne Bourquin, Syracuse, N.Y.
Gladys Branegan, Bozeman, Mont.
Jean Brodie, Nashville, Tenn.
Margaret Hessler Brooks, Chicago, Ill.
Blanche E. Brown, Danbury, Conn.
Mrs. Louise M. Brown, Washington, D.C.
Olga P. Brucher, Ithaca, N.Y.
†Mrs. Mary de Garmo Bryan, New York, N.Y.
Marjorie E. Burr, Manchester, Conn.
Anna de Planter Bowes, Harrisburg, Pa.
H. C. Cameron, Morgantown, W. Va.
Janet L. Cameron, Blacksburg, Va.
H. Louise Campbell, New York, N.Y.
Pearl S. Camstra, Watkinsville, Ga.
G. Carlson, Minneapolis, Minn.
Edna M. Caton, Harrisburg, Pa.
Eleanor F. Chase, Amesbury, Mass.
Agnes K. Clarke, Alfred, N.Y.
Helen Clarke, Winter Park, Fla.
Jessie G. Cole, Albany, N.Y.
†Lenna F. Cooper, New York, N.Y.
H. W. Cruise, Menominee, Wis.
Mary Dahnke, Chicago, Ill.

**Participated by being present at the dinner or in some other way*
†Members of the Committee

Linagail Darling, Brooklyn, N.Y.
Dorothy De Hart, New York, N.Y.
Marie Dohm, New York, N.Y.
Bernice Dodge, Chicago, Ill.
Laura Drummond, State College, Pa.
Jessie E. Duncan, Bronx, N.Y.
Alice Edwards, Washington, D.C.
Bertha B. Edwards, Portland, Oreg.
Margaret Edwards, Greensboro, N.C.
Elizabeth Ellis, Durham, N.H.
Mrs. Casa Emeilos, New York, N.Y.
Dorothy Engleman, Narrowsburg, N.Y.
Rachel M. Fabrick, Woodside, N.Y.
Emma E. Feeney, Brooklyn, N.Y.
Faith Fenton, Ithaca, N.Y.
Genevieve Fisher, Ames, Iowa
Natalie K. Fitch, New York, N.Y.
Henrietta Fleck, Newark, Del.
M. M. Fotheringham, Buffalo, N.Y.
Anne Franfelder, Nazareth, Pa.
Lucille G. French, New Medford, Mass.
Irma L. Gamble, Peoria, Ill.
Alice M. Garman, Hamden, Conn.
Dolores Garrett, Jersey City, N.J.
Miriam Garrison, Amherst, Mass.
Alma L. Garvin, Columbus, Ohio
Beatrice J. Geiger, Cedar Falls, Iowa
Margaret S. Gillam, New York, N.Y.
Lucy H. Gillett, New York, N.Y.
Cora Gray, Salisbury, N.C.
Eleanor V. Green, Flushing, N.Y.
†Elizabeth Guilford, New York, N.Y.
Mrs. Charles Gus, Brooklyn, N.Y.
Faye I. Hamilton, Newark, N.J.
Clara Hesslock, Milledgeville, Ga.
Desdemona Heinrich, New York, N.Y.
Betsy Helburn, Bronx, N.Y.
Marjorie M. Heseltine, Washington, D.C.
Hazel D. Higgins, Lewiston, Maine
Geraldine G. Hill, New York, N.Y.
Ada A. Hillier, South Bend, Ind.
Frances L. Hoag, Philadelphia, Pa.
Sarah H. Holmes, New York, N.Y.
Helen Hubbell, New Haven, Conn.
Mary P. Huddleson, New Canaan, Conn.
Mrs. Lauretta P. James, West Chester, Pa.
Florence Joffe, Brooklyn, N.Y.
Florence Johnston, Brooklyn, N.Y.
Lucy E. Jones, Newark, N.J.
Mrs. Ida Jean Kain, Manhasset, N.Y.
Helen B. Kay, New York, N.Y.
Sara Kerr, Ithaca, N.Y.
Dorothy W. Kirk, New York, N.Y.
Martha M. Kramer, Peiping, China
Lan-Chen Kung, Peiping, China
Amalia Lautz, Fredericksburg, Pa.
Louise L'Engle, Ames, Iowa
V. Lukofsky, Bronx, N.Y.
M. E. MacLean, Johnson, Vt.
†Grace MacLeod, New York, N.Y.
Mrs. E. A. Martin, Chicago, Ill.
Mrs. J. H. Martin, Durham, N.C.
Susan Mathews, Athens, Ga.
Florence McAllister, Mt. Vernon, N.Y.
Mary McCormick, Albany, N.Y.
J. McCreery, Lubbock, Tex.
Esther McGinnis, Minneapolis, Minn.
Wylie B. McNeal, St. Paul, Minn.
†Adeline R. Missal, Bristol, Conn.
Day Monroe, Washington, D.C.
Helen Monsch, Ithaca, N.Y.
Eleanor B. Moorland, Morgantown, W. Va.
Edith Swan Morey, Swarthmore, Pa.

Hazel Munsell, New York, N.Y.
†Pauline Murrah, New York, N.Y.
Eleanor Nance, Ithaca, N.Y.
E. C. Nickerson, Hartford, Conn.
Mary W. Northrop, Seattle, Wash.
Marie O'Donahoe, Bronx, N.Y.
Frances Alida Pattee, Mt. Vernon, N.Y.
Ina Padgett, State College, Pa.
Joseph Pascal, M.D., New York, N.Y.
Esther Phipard, Washington, D.C.
Martha Pittman, Manhattan, Kans.
Henrietta Pribnow, Philadelphia, Pa.
Ellen Reed, Sault Ste. Marie, Ontario, Canada
Gladys H. Reeha, Anaheim, Calif.
Grace Reeves, New York, N.Y.
Catharine Reigart, Yonkers, N.Y.
Anna M. Renigh, Elizabeth, N.J.
Martha Rogers, Washington, D.C.
†Elda Robb, Philadelphia, Pa.
Mrs. Barbara Robson, Berkeley, Calif.
Hannah Honeywell Rose, Windsor, Conn.
Katharine Roy, Saratoga, N.Y.
Deborah M. Russell, Framingham, Mass.
Margaret P. Sandals, Tallahassee, Fla.
Marie Sayles, Flint, Mich.
Clyde B. Schuman, New York, N.Y.
Naomi Schnelier, Elmhurst, N.Y.
Mary L. Shapiro, New York, N.Y.
Bess Smenner, Staten Island, N.Y.
Daisy M. Smith, Jenkintown, Pa.
Mrs. Helen Smith, Walton, N.Y.
Emma R. Southworth, Troy, N.Y.
Gertrude T. Spitz, Brookline, Mass.
Phyllis K. Sprague, State College, Pa.
Helen Stacey, New York, N.Y.
Dorothy M. Stephens, New York, N.Y.
Hazel Stiebeling, Washington, D.C.
Harriet Stone, Newark, N.J.
†Clara Mae Taylor, New York, N.Y.
E. M. Thompson, Tucson, Ariz.
M. E. Thompson, New York, N.Y.
Doris H. Tisdale, New York, N.Y.
C. P. Townsend, Greenwich, N.Y.
Eunice M. True, Berea, Ky.
Gertrude M. True, Arlington, Va.
Tumbridge, Brooklyn, N.Y.
Rhoda A. Tyler, Valhalla, N.Y.
Ella McC. Vahlteich, Edgewater, N.J.
Lenore Van der Sloot, New York, N.Y.
Alice W. Van Dyke, New York, N.Y.
Mary E. Walton, New Haven, Conn.
Gladys J. Ward, Urbana, Ill.
Sarah Jane Weber, New York, N.Y.
Margaret M. Weeks, Lubbock, Tex.
Blanche Weidman, New York, N.Y.
Lucille Welch, Sutzton, Pa.
R. E. Wertz, New York, N.Y.
Martha Westfall, Brooklyn, N.Y.
Margaret Whittemore, Kingston, R.I.
Eustis Wightman, Woodbury, Conn.
Dorothy E. Williams, Knoxville, Tenn.
Jet C. Winters, Austin, Texas
Mrs. K. C. Wiseley, New York, N.Y.
Mrs. B. S. W. Worsham, Jackson Heights, N.Y.
Mrs. James W. Wuetz, San Francisco, Calif.

INDEX